Empty Arms: A Heavy Load to Carry

Dorothy Donham

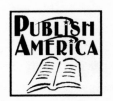
PUBLISH AMERICA

PublishAmerica
Baltimore

First printing

ISBN: 1-4137-5090-7
PUBLISHED BY PUBLISHAMERICA, LLLP
www.publishamerica.com
Baltimore

Printed in the United States of America

Acknowledgments

First and foremost, I would like to thank God for giving me the most unbelievable miracles of my life—my children. They came to us under extraordinary circumstances. Even when I felt abandoned and alone in my heartache, I was not. God was quietly there holding me in His loving hands. Without Him, my trial would have never turned into triumph.

To my husband, Jody, words cannot express the love in my heart for you as you stood by my side supporting me through the most difficult time in my life. You wiped my tears, prayed with me, and encouraged me. You were always willing to go the extra mile no matter what craziness I had thought up for us to try. You are the love of my life and I am forever grateful that God placed you in my life. I love you!

To my children, you are the miracles of my life. You have opened places in my heart that I never knew existed. The love that flows from me to you is immeasurable. I thank God daily for you and for the joy and healing you have brought to me. I love you, my darlings.

To my family, thank you all so much for the fervent prayers that you prayed in our behalf. I believe you reached the throne room of God, making a way for Hope and Jayden to be sent to us. Each of you did something that touched us in a special way. Your considerate actions ranged from Mom asking every person she met to pray we would have a child, to Deanna supporting and comforting me during childbirth. Not to mention every other thoughtful deed from each one of you in between. I feel so blessed to be a part of this family that God gave me. I love you all.

To my friends and church family, I would have never made it without you. All of the lunches that were interrupted by tears, all of the three and four hour phone calls, all of the crazy fertility tricks tried and shared, and finally, a baby shower fit for royalty—thank you Christy, Heather and Deanna. You were my towers of strength and my much-needed sounding board. To all of my other friends and coworkers at the Mary Babb Randolph Cancer Center, who gave me support during my infertility and in-vitro fertilization attempt, it meant the world to me. I feel so fortunate to have my life surrounded by such extraordinary human beings. I love you all.

To Rev. Null, thank you for yielding to God's voice and humbly delivering His word to me. I clung to that promise. It was all that I had left to hold onto and it got me through my hardest times. You'll never know how much that meant to me. You hold a special place in our hearts.

To Dr. Yalcinkaya, Dr. Olar, Dr. Burns, Cherese, and all of the staff who cared for us at Charleston Area Medical Center, I could never thank you enough for the superb care we received. The professionalism each of you displayed intermingled with love and compassion far exceeded the norm. It was because of you, with God's help, that we have our miracle baby. We are forever indebted to you for the gift we have been blessed with. May God richly bless each one of you.

To Dr. Hembree, thank you for your care, concern, and guidance during this journey. I was thrilled and honored that you were able to be present and deliver our miracle safely into the world. You made difficult and uncertain times a little easier for us. You have been more than a physician to us—you have been a friend.

Introduction

A mirror casts an honest reflection. It reveals both beautiful and unattractive truths. Just as the mirror, our lives reflect who we are, where we have been, and what we believe.

This journal is my reflection. It's a story of trial to triumph while gaining a renewed faith in the end. Most of all it's my story, framing the handiwork of God as He performed a miracle in my life.

I started this journal as a keepsake for my unborn angel, and then continued it as an outlet for overwhelming emotions. It was therapeutic, as I would tap away at my computer for hours on end, pouring out the heartache that was building up inside of me. My entries were quite personal and candid, sometimes seemingly irrational.

Now looking in hindsight, I can clearly see where God has brought me. In some cases, I can see why I had to travel the paths that I did. Had I been privileged to the "bigger picture" from the beginning, I would have taken a different journey. I'm thankful I didn't—I wouldn't be the person I am today. God never left my side, even though I felt at times He had abandoned me. He watched over me and lovingly cared for me as I struggled through my ordeal. In the end, I got to know God differently as I witnessed His sovereignty and miracle-working power in my life. I may not have all of the answers from my struggle, but I have found myself in a wonderful place that otherwise I may have never been.

There are over six million women dealing with infertility today. Infertility does not discriminate. It doesn't matter how well planned your life is, what church you attend, or how long you put your faith in God. I felt that as a child of God, I should have been exempt from this pain. I quickly learned that I am human and therefore I am prone to suffer things of this flesh. I was not exempt from this affliction.

The subject of infertility is often taboo because of the private aspect of our lives that it involves. We often are embarrassed or feel that we have done something wrong to cause this to happen. Infertility then becomes an excruciating secret that can destroy you from the inside out.

There is hope within the hurting. I know because I have been there. I could not have made it without my faith and trust in the Lord. I clung to His word. Psalms 119:105 states, "Thy word is a lamp unto my feet and a light unto my path." Even though I stumbled over what seemed to be impassable obstacles, I learned to follow God's direction and to trust Him when things were not clear. That is why I decided to share our story.

My prayer is that the contents of this journal will touch the life of someone, giving hope and encouragement to them as they fight the same battles I once did. I hope it provides insight to someone who has a family member or friend that struggles with infertility, because it relays some of the common feelings and hardships often experienced. I pray that God touches that person's life the way He touched mine.

September 22, 1997

To my precious little one,

I have dreamed of you for quite some time now. For as long as I can remember, I've had a strong maternal instinct, wanting to share my love with something that belonged to me. Growing up, I fantasized about what my baby would look like and what it would be like caring for something so special and unique.

After I met your daddy, I still fantasized about you. Every time we saw a child we compared features and talked about how they would look like yours. When we saw chubby cheeks, blond curly hair, or just an adorably plump baby, we would say, "That's what our baby is going to look like!" We spent lots of time creating distinctive names and making decisions about how we would raise you before you were even a reality.

We are not the only ones thinking about your arrival. You have four wonderful grandparents and five great-grandparents impatiently waiting! They always ask us when they can expect you and why it is taking so long for your arrival. They are all so very anxious to meet you and shower you with their love.

So you see, precious one, you have been wanted for a very long time. Almost my whole lifetime! When you do finally come into this world you will have lots of love, warmth and security waiting for you.

After your daddy and I got married, people asked us when we would have a baby. I would reply matter-of-factly, "When it happens, it does. If it doesn't right now, that's fine, too. We haven't had a deep desire for a baby yet." But I stand corrected, dear one.

When I made the decision to start this journal now, before I even carry you in my womb, I have learned that I always had a very deep desire and longing for you in my life. I will always want you to know as you grow inside of me, and throughout your life, that you were wanted before you even came to "be."

On August 4th, 1997, I had a doctor's appointment, my annual check-up. I had experienced some difficulties with my health since my previous visit, so I prepared a lot of questions that day for the doctor. She had some answers to those questions. Answers that I was not prepared to hear. As I listened to her in that confined, sterile environment, I felt as if I had a tornado within my being, whirling around my emotions. Failure, confusion, anger, and so much more than words could even describe. If these feelings would have been set free at that time I am convinced they could have leveled the tri-state area! You wonder why such devastation and destruction was inside of me? It was because my doctor told me I might never have you.

In a very professional and reassuring tone the doctor explained that my body was not working correctly to produce a baby. When the time came there would be a lot of doctor visits, tests, medications, and procedures. This didn't sound like an appealing future. I was just twenty-four years old and had a relatively benign history. I couldn't imagine why this had to happen—especially to me! After I composed myself I decided that I would do whatever it took to bring you into this world.

That day I went home to your daddy with my spirit broken. I tried to put on the most confident, unaffected voice that I could muster while telling him what the doctor had said. Even though I believe he saw right through my charade, he was entirely untouched. Your daddy is very strong. It seems that an earthquake of the largest magnitude doesn't affect him. I am so glad of that because I am sensitive to even the smallest vibrations.

Your daddy went about his day and I rushed right out to the mall to buy a book on infertility. Infertility felt like such a "dirty" word. I took cover and watched over my shoulder making sure no one I knew saw me browsing the section in the bookstore. I finally found one and escaped the bookstore unseen. I read the whole thing cover to cover in less than twenty-four hours. I felt better after educating myself some, but deep down inside, I had a gnawing feeling. I prayed about it a lot and read 1 Samuel several times in the Bible. It was comforting to read how Hannah struggled before the Lord and how He honored her prayers by blessing her with a son.

I then prayed even more and allowed God to help me carry some of the load. I made plans to start the fertility testing at the beginning of the new year and decided that we would just go from there.

On August 31, 1997, just twenty-seven days after the visit with my doctor, we had a guest speaker at our church. Rev. Terry Null preached a powerful message that night. The Lord's presence encompassed that service. The minister talked about how Elizabeth was barren and how an angel spoke to her husband and told him that they would have a son. I sat in the pew with tears streaming down my cheeks because of the recent news I'd received regarding my condition.

Rev. Null led an altar call and I went up to the platform as usual to play my keyboard. He told the congregation, "In order to receive that 'thing' in your life that you have been praying for, you will have to start praising God with your whole heart." He told us that if we praised God and did not dwell in our situations, God would honor us and give us the miracle that we needed. He then stopped the musicians and said that he felt that someone on the platform needed the opportunity to pray. So the musicians prayed and the spirit of the Lord just flooded that place! It was overwhelming. I received a touch from God that night like no other. I was worrying about several different situations. I started to feel a peace about these things and a healing started deep within me. Not just physically, but spiritually and emotionally too. A lot of negativity that I had bottled up flowed out of me that night.

While I was praying, Rev. Null came over and placed his hands on my temples. He didn't say anything special, and then he just walked away. A short time later, as we continued to pray, Rev. Null came a second time and prayed with me. This time I remember two phrases that he prayed over me that I believe came straight from God: "So be it. So let it be done." And, "Trust me. Just trust me." Those words thundered in my ears and went straight through me like lightening bolts! Even though I was praying for many different things that night, I knew right then the one thing he was speaking of. It was your existence.

As soon as service was dismissed, Rev. Null came over to talk with me. He said, "You have been praying for many things for a long time."

I confirmed that I had. Through tear-clouded eyes I confided in him by pouring out the contents of my troubled heart. I told him about all of the illness in our family, my unhappiness with my job, and that I had received a "bad report" from a doctor. These were among many other things that had been going on.

He looked directly into my eyes and said, "God has heard your prayers. This is the fourth time that God has spoken to me about a barren woman. He told me that you will conceive a baby." He went on to tell me, "One of the other three women was told that under no circumstance could she bare a child. Today she has a son!"

With tears racing down my already chapped face, I said with a choked voice, "But I want my mother healed."

And he replied, "Yes, but God is giving you life."

That night we teased your daddy and grandparents about the prophecy I had received. We happily entertained the thought of your arrival and elevated everyone's anticipation of you. I feel like I got a word straight from God through a humble minister who lent himself as a willing messenger.

After that night I felt a tremendous change occur inside of me. I was able to give the whole thing over to God for Him to control. I had not yet felt the need to begin the testing my doctor recommended, but I did feel the need to start this journal. I wanted something I could share with you to tell you that you are a priceless gift from God that was promised to your daddy and me.

Even though you have not been sent to me yet, I believe that you are waiting in heaven for the perfect time to come and live with

Mommy and Daddy. I believe that you are hand-picked by God to be our special little angel. I am watching the calendar endlessly until we learn of your impending arrival into this world.

With a lifetime of love,

Mommy

March 15, 1998

To my dear child,

It has been a long six months since I've written an entry in this journal. We have taken a wild ride on this emotional roller coaster of fertility treatments. There have been a lot of unexpected twists and turns along the way. Just when we would climb to the top of a situation and feel like we were making progress, we would plummet down the other side again with our hearts in our throats. My desire has now turned into desperation.

Last December, I decided to start the testing that my doctor recommended for me. I had to endure blood tests, x-rays, and humiliating procedures. Not to mention all of the probing questions about my personal life and being put on display for impersonal strangers to invade. I remember one particular test that was so painful, I just lay helplessly on the table and cried. I prayed silently that God would take away the discomfort, the testing, and the problems. Unfortunately, there are things in life that we have to face whether it suits us or not. Some situations may be quite painful, but God has always proved faithful.

I survived the initial testing. I felt like a soldier fresh out of boot camp! Now it was time to go to war—with fertility drugs. I started my first cycle in January, 1998. I wasn't sure what to expect. I talked to a pharmacist and my doctor. I read all of the literature I could find, but I still had an uneasy feeling of the unknown.

After a major letdown, the first month came and went with no results except some newly acquired hot flashes. What an understatement! There were times that I felt like I was experiencing spontaneous combustion! Some days I would have liked to trade the little fan in my purse for a fire extinguisher.

The funny part of it is that your Grammy is going through menopause and we had our share of hot flashes together. I don't think that I will ever forget that blustery January day at the bank window. We had a simultaneous hot flash in the car and just about exploded! We were peeling each other's coats off and rolling down the windows while we attempted to fan ourselves. The air conditioner just couldn't blow enough cool air! Snow belted in the open windows on our sweat-beaded faces as both of us panted and laughed at the same time. What a sight we were. I will never forget the puzzled look on the bank tellers' faces. I am sure they will never forget us, either.

I read more about the medication I was taking. I was upset when I read that if it didn't work in the first cycle, chances were low that it would be effective in following attempts. I felt like all of the efforts I was making were in vain. All of the temperature charts, medications, blood tests, and ultra sounds were for nothing. I had a real pity party for myself that day. God straightened out my attitude pretty fast. He gave me a promise that He will keep. God cannot lie and He is faithful. This is what I have held on to for the past few months and the only reason why I have kept my sanity during this time.

At the end of my second cycle I had some changes. Every day, sometimes several times a day, I would get my calendar out and count … and count … and count. Could it be? I was late! My heart thumped so wildly that I thought it would leap right out of my chest! This had happened many times before and I faced great disappointment, but this time I was on fertility drugs. There was hope. I didn't say much to anyone, not even your daddy. Then after a few more days, I nonchalantly let him know that I may need a pregnancy test. I believe he may have been just as excited as I was.

Several days later I was back at the hospital working in the pediatric step-down unit. I went to the lab to have my blood drawn again. They told me that my results would take about an hour and a half. That was the longest hour of my life. I was so glad to have work to return to because it kept me busy. Every time I thought about it I trembled with the pure thrill of the thought that you could be coming into our lives. My hands shook so badly I could hardly accomplish anything. My heart raced as my emotions stirred—I just knew this was it! I spent most of the hour and a half wait planning how I would tell your daddy. What an occasion!

Two-thirty p.m., finally! Time to call the lab. I sat at the desk almost shivering with glee. I was so out of breath I could hardly mutter my name when the lab tech answered the phone. She searched for my results. The tapping of the keyboard echoed in my ears competing with the sound of my pulse as she typed the information into the computer. I thought I would pass out with anticipation before she could tell me the result!

"Mrs. Donham, I have your result right here. It is less than three—it is negative."

At that moment the whole world stopped around me. I could see the busy day moving in its usual chaotic fashion, but I couldn't hear it. I don't even think I drew another breath until I finally managed a weak, "Thank you." The telephone dropped from my limp hand to the desk. I was paralyzed with grief. My body was numb from the adrenalin I had built up as it surged through my veins only moments before. I know that my face drained to a ghostly white color because another nurse rushed over to me asking if I was OK. I told her yes, and then scrambled for the bathroom where I sobbed until the tears would no longer flow.

It was pretty tough to get through that day, promise or no promise. With each passing day that I grew even later I became more bitter and angry with my body. I could not control this thing, but it sure had control of me. At the end of every cycle it was like facing a death. I would mourn over what had not happened and then would begin to look ahead for hope in the next cycle. This repeated month after month.

Babies! Babies! Babies! Everyone around me has been getting pregnant or having babies. Invitations to baby showers come at record speed and have created another obstacle for me. The time came for my sister-in-law's baby shower. I felt so awkward as I walked through the door. I literally felt like I had a neon sign above my head flashing "infertile" and "failure." I sat down at the table with the family and did all I could do to restrain the tears. It was difficult to see the baby gifts and hear all of the comments. I just wanted to die. I couldn't hide from the hopeless emptiness I fought inside of me. I left within an hour. I couldn't stand anymore of this private hell I lived in.

Then there were the girls at work. It seemed as though every week another one would announce that she was pregnant. One morning while we sat in the report room, another coworker announced that she, too, was pregnant. I got a few pitiful looks from friends that knew how I secretly longed for a child. It seemed like I was immediately on center stage as everyone stared at me to see how I would react. I put on the biggest smile I could configure and gave her all of the appropriate congratulations. All the while I felt like someone was shredding my inner self as it was being ripped apart piece by piece. It hurt so badly.

Eleven days had passed before my body started working correctly again, thus starting my third cycle on the fertility drugs. Now we have more tests to determine if we need an alternative course of therapy after this attempt.

Some days I have a lot of faith. Some days I feel like I am the biggest failure that ever walked the earth. As long as I keep my eyes on God and you, my goal, I will make it. I am learning patience through all of this and the meaning of "God's timing is not our own." After God blesses me with you, my miracle, I know that I will be a different person for standing up in the face of adversity and making it through. I also know that someday as I cradle you in my arms, my love for you will not be the same as most mothers. I will not only have my desire satisfied, but also a prophecy fulfilled from God. I will be holding the blessing of a miracle—you! Although right now I have to face a lot of hurt and pain, it will be worth every second of the agony just to have you.

I love you my sweet desire,

Mommy

March 23, 1998

To my sweet child,

My heart is longing for you today. My womb aches to carry you. It feels like eternity has come and gone and we still don't have you. I tried to cry so that I could empty some of these emotions, but I just didn't have the strength in me. This has been one of the greatest challenges that I have faced in my life.

Friday, March 20, 1998 (your Grammy's 51st birthday), I had an ultrasound performed. Dr H. wanted to check for developing follicles in my ovaries. Your daddy and I were so excited. It almost felt like we were going to get a glimpse of you today. We watched the screen as she scanned my womb. We were not able to visualize my right ovary due to a full bladder. She then found my left ovary and said, "Happy Easter, you laid an egg!" We found several follicles developing there, but one in particular was ready to "pop." We were absolutely elated! It seemed like I would finally be carrying you.

Even though we wouldn't find out if I would become pregnant for another few weeks, no one could wipe the smiles off of our faces that day. We were so giddy that whole night. Nothing could tame our excitement of the progress we had made. For once it finally felt like we would have a chance at parenthood.

I don't know how I am going to make it to the end of the month. My mind has been held hostage. Every time I promise myself that I won't dwell in this, I drown myself in desperation again.

Today at work I took another emotional blow. Yet another coworker announced that she is pregnant. I was genuinely happy for her, but I started to feel myself sink deep inside. If that was not enough, I spent the whole day with a pregnant nurse in the step-down unit. I felt the little bit of faith and hope that I had built up turn into doubt and misery with each congratulation and inquiry that came her way. I started to think, *What makes this cycle any different from the others? I'll never become pregnant.* I feel so guilty because I know others deserve all of this attention. I just wish I could separate myself from it. It is quite a lonely place to be.

I know that you are promised to me. I am just so impatient. It seems like something so wonderful will never happen to me. I feel like I have lost the ability to trust. I have trusted God to deliver His promise, I have trusted the doctors to order the correct procedures and medications, and I have trusted the medications to work properly. And I still don't have you. I think about you every waking moment and I daydream of the time we find out that we are expecting you. It just seems so unimaginable! It is comforting to know that someday I will be able to look back on this time in my life, read this journal, hold you close, and say to myself, "It's over and I made it through."

As always, I am anxiously and impatiently waiting for you. I love you so much already and I don't even have you yet. Just thinking of how it is going to be, having you in our lives, makes my heart flutter with anticipation and excitement!

With all my love always,
Mommy

April 4, 1998

To my precious little child,

I face another difficult milestone today. Today I realize that you will not be arriving in 1998. This morning I awoke to the painful realization that my new cycle had started. I cried for hours. I lay helplessly in bed until your daddy came home from work. In my emotional frailty I couldn't make myself get out of bed. I just didn't know what to do.

I feel like I am in my own isolated little world that not even prayer can penetrate. I know how very wrong that statement is, but the fact does not change how I feel.

This will be an emotionally challenging week for certain. My expectations have been rising to unbelievable levels. I have taken my share of hard falls lately and I am starting to feel quite battered. I have just about lost touch with life because I have surrounded myself with the obsession of you.

I know I have to make some changes now before my sanity slips away. I have to change my obsession into dedication, a pattern that will be hard to break. My longing to be a mother to you is so intense that it gets very difficult to separate these feelings. Today I have decided to set some new goals.

Instead of agonizing every month, I will have faith and trust in God for His perfect will and timing for our lives. I will not allow negative thoughts to overpower my positive thoughts. I will continue to have high expectations, believing that one day they will be fulfilled. I will continue to pray each day about you even if it feels like my prayers are not getting past the ceiling. I will not be defeated, but determined. I will use this trial to my advantage and become strong and lean totally on God. I will continue to give thanks and praise to God no matter the outcome of my day.

I am dedicating myself to having you. No matter how high the cost, I want you. I will have you! It may not be my perfect plan, but it will be God's perfect plan. How wonderful it will be for you to know that you are God's masterpiece and that He designed you to custom fit His perfect plan for our lives. That truly excites me and comforts my heart. I love you and I will not stop until I get you. You may not be coming as soon as we had wished, but I know that you are on the way. For some reason God has us riding along the scenic route. I am sure that as we travel the road of life, we will pass some beautiful things, and I am sure we will have our share of bumpy roads, too. Then our understanding will be enlightened as to why you were not sent to us sooner.

Until it is time, sweet baby, dance with the angels, sparkle with the stars, float on fluffy clouds, and know that Mommy and Daddy love you and are yearning for you. We will always have an empty place in our lives until you fill the void. We will continue to watch the heavens and dream of you every night until God sends us our precious little angel of love—you!

I love you,
Mommy

May 12, 1998

To my cherished little treasure,

So much has happened since I last wrote to you, my sweet child. God has this in His hands because I have given Him control. He knows our overwhelming desire for you, and I know He will send you to us according to His perfect will and timing.

I have faced some very difficult things in the past month. The pressure has been greater than at any other time. I feel as if I have a heavy weight crushing my heart as it struggles to beat on. Another mark in this journey has been made. Easter. At the beginning of my treatments I looked hopefully ahead in my calendar and marked Easter. All of my fertility drugs would be completed by that time and I knew I would surely be pregnant by Easter. Unfortunately, I was not. I left church early, retreating to my car as I tried to deal with my sorrow. Again, I cried all day. It was one of the more painful days that I have had, but I made it through.

We did have a bit of joyful news this past month. Your cousin Nathan "Mitchell" Donham was born to your Uncle Shawn and Aunt Tracy. I remember going to visit them and just gazing at his perfect little face. He was absolutely adorable! I couldn't help but think that could be me holding you. I also thought how much you would most likely look like him. So preciously plump, blondish hair, and the cutest little nose! Oh, how it made me ache for you.

Yet another cycle has started. I called my physician and asked if I could now be referred to a fertility specialist. The arrangements are being made, but I have not been able to see him yet. I asked if I could take another cycle of fertility drugs just so I could feel like we were doing something while waiting to see Dr. T. I just couldn't let this month go by wasting valuable time. So now we wait and pray that this is the month God answers our prayers.

The ironic thing is, this could be the very month you do come to us. On Friday, May 8th, we had a special youth service hosting several different churches. Guess who was there. Rev. Null. We had an awesome service. Rev. Null called me over and the ministers prayed for me once again. I could really feel something happening! I went back to my keyboard and began playing again, but still feeling very moved within. Rev. Null came over and laid his hands on top of mine and said, "Stop with all of your questioning. You need to consider some other pathways or options." Then he said it. The dreaded word that I feared and was hiding from. He just blurted it out—Adoption! I just about fainted. That word was not part of my vocabulary. Especially when applying it to me!

He went on to say that he received a phone call the night before from a minister in Tennessee. He told Rev. Null that there is a young lady, a college student, who is in need. She is pregnant and needs help. She and her boyfriend are unable to provide the baby with the love, attention and finances that it will need. She loves this child so much that she wants to give it to a loving Christian couple who will care for this precious little life as their very own. Rev. Null asked your daddy and me to pray earnestly about the situation and consider adopting the child when it is born.

I was absolutely blown away! I had this stupid smile on my face and just nodded my head to everything Rev. Null said. He probably thought that I was thinking he was a lunatic by my reactions. I was just flabbergasted! To top it off, Rev. Null had to leave church early that night to go out of town. Therefore, I was unable to speak with him further regarding the situation.

That night, I could hardly talk without being extremely emotional. I couldn't sleep. It raced through my mind every second from the moment it spilled from Rev. Null's lips. Your daddy and I talked about it that night and prayed. He made it sound so perfect, so right, but I was still confused. Rev. Null told me not to question and then he threw this in front of me. I had questions!

Will I love this child the same? Will this child love me? Will this child resent us? Is this God's will? Is this child you—the one we have been praying for so long? I have to honestly say that at this time most of those questions are still unanswered and may remain that way for quite some time. Only God knows the answers.

I also have to admit that I am hung up on the biological thing. We spent so much time dreaming of what our baby will look like. Whose smile will you have? Will you be short or tall? Will you have Mommy's eyes or Daddy's chin? I also did my share of fantasizing about what it will be like to carry you in my womb, watching my tummy grow, and to feel you kick inside of me. Will we ever experience these things? I don't know. They have to be in God's perfect plan for our lives.

What a struggle! Ugh! There is a part of me that wants to jump in the car and head for this sweet little child. Another part of me wants to restrain myself to wait for a pregnancy. But will it happen? If it does, will it even be anytime soon? What pain and agony this has brought to my heart. If we choose this baby, is it really you? Could God have sent your precious little soul to someone else just so that we may trust Him more? Know this, we will be in God's will whatever decision is made. We are praying that if this is truly God's will for our lives, the doors will remain open and we'll get through without complications. If it is not God's will, we pray that God shuts the door and another couple is blessed with this fragile little miracle. So wherever God leads, it will not be a mistake.

On Monday evening, around 11:30 p.m., we received a call from Rev. Null. He had more information for us about this mixed blessing. He was able to provide details about the situation that put our minds at ease. I actually got extremely excited. In fact, so excited that I was calling people in the middle of the night getting them out of bed to tell them about our fantastic news. We were going to proceed with the adoption!

Was God giving peace to my heart? Could this be it? He told us that we would be receiving a phone call from the pastor in Tennessee that was taking care of the adoption. He would provide us with more information.

We do know that the baby is due June 10th. We don't know the sex of the baby yet, but I am going to try to find out. We have so much to do and a little less than a month to do it all in. I am scared stiff. I just want to be doing the right thing and remain in God's will. We have to remodel the downstairs (we thought we would have 9 months to do that in!), we have to obtain necessities for the baby, contact the appropriate people, and make arrangements at work. Unbelievable!

We have had an uncountable amount of support through this and numerous people praying along with us for God's will. Dear child, please know that whatever package God sends you in, whatever state you are born in, and no matter what woman gives birth to you, you will be ours. We will love you unconditionally. The word "biological" will not be used in our home. You will not need our genetic make-up to be loved or cared for because you were wanted for so long, angel.

Even though things are moving toward adoption, I still get the feeling I will become pregnant someday. Last night, I had a vision. We were called to a prayer meeting at the church and naturally I was praying for you and this situation. I found myself walking down a bright white corridor and I saw Jesus on His throne. I didn't see His face, just a brilliantly illuminated figure holding an infant. The child was wrapped in a blue blanket and I could not see its face. He leaned over and handed me the baby.

I feel like that was you. I believe that you are being cradled safely in the arms of God right now. I don't know what route you will come to us, but I do feel that it will be soon.

It could be just a few weeks until we cradle our heaven-sent blessing in our arms, or it may be a few years. God moves mysteriously. We love you and long for you, our sweet child.

With a yearning heart full of love,

Mommy

May 22, 1998

To my dear precious love,

Well, my dear love, I stand disappointed, but not devastated. In fact, maybe somewhat encouraged.

After an intense emotion-tangling week, we have learned part of God's plan and are now moving in His will. After a week of calling four lawyers (in three states), making preparations at work and with family, arranging for a contractor to remodel, and finally, shopping for a crib, we got our answer.

On Friday, May 15th, around midnight, we received a phone call from the pastor in Tennessee. He called to tell us that the first couple that was contacted by the birth mother had changed their minds and now decided, "Yes." They wanted to adopt the unborn infant. It was only one week to the day that we were asked to take the child. I felt like we had been dealing with this for a year! My heart sank as I listened to your daddy's end of the conversation. I could tell that we had lost our chance at this opportunity. The amazing thing is that I did not and have not cried over it. We are in God's will.

The next day we made all of the necessary phone calls to family, friends and employers to notify them of the abrupt change in plans. It hurt a little, but still there was also an underlying sense of relief that came.

It has now been another week since we learned we would not be adopting this child. I have thought about it off and on, but my focus is back to you again. I called my physician and completed the arrangements to see a specialist on June 1st. I am very eager to make this next step. I know that you will be coming to us soon. I just feel it within me!

I have viewed the most recent events as a test from God. I feel like He was challenging us to see if we would be submissive to His will and not our will. I also feel like He wanted to see if we would truly lean on Him and give Him complete control, no matter what the situation. I don't know if it's because we will face some great thing in the future, or if you will still come to us by adoption. What I do know is that we passed the test. That soothes my heart.

I have to admit that as we were rushing around like mad people making plans, I felt a certain emptiness within my soul. I just knew it was not going to happen yet. I didn't want to let that feeling put a damper on my excitement, though. It was very thrilling to finally be planning for our child. I got a good taste of what it is going to be like to plan for your arrival. Only this time, I will be able to savor every moment!

I love you my adored little one,

Mommy

June 24, 1998

To my dearest little one,

It has been one month and two days since I wrote you last, sweet child. I cannot describe to you the way I am feeling. I have so many mixed emotions. It seems like things have hit an all-time low and when I feel like it can't get worse—it does. I have a lot of catching up to do since my last entry in your journal. My heart has been so heavy and broken. I have had a difficult time making myself sit down and do this.

On June 1st, we had our appointment with our fertility specialist. What a grueling experience! The morning of our appointment was nerve-wracking. We arrived to a crowded waiting room where we sat for two long hours. The whole time I had an awful feeling of nausea spill over me. I couldn't sit still and I certainly couldn't concentrate on a magazine. All of the "what ifs" gushed through my weary mind. I felt like I was losing my mind. I don't think your daddy was doing much better.

After our long unexpected wait (apparently two emergency cases came in before us), we made it to an examination room. The nurse greeted us as she settled us in. She was very gentle and kind. Short of having white hair, she felt like the all-American grandmother. Her love and compassion radiated about her as she did her work. Then we got to meet our doctor. Dr. T. whisked through the exam room door with his head down, hand protruded, and he somehow managed to shake both of ours in the process of mumbling his name. I could tell this would be an interesting experience at best.

Dr. T. asked some general questions about our past medical

history without much apparent concern. I felt like we were being "processed" through our time of turmoil. I had to restrain myself from running out of the room. I didn't know if I could keep myself composed to get through this. Next he decided that he needed to do a head-to-toe exam—and that he did! I was totally unsuspecting of what he had in mind and it was very humiliating. Before I even knew what happened, I found my arm above my head, my gown opened, and a breast exam being performed. His same cool, unaffected mannerism that was present in his questioning was displayed during the exam, too. To add to the degrading circumstance, he had a few rude remarks to make about my body. Namely my big feet! I felt like shoving them down his throat. I certainly was in the position to do just that. I just kept telling myself that he was only trying to lighten up the situation by cracking a joke, although at my expense.

Except for some of my past medical history with my cycles, he found my physical exam normal. That was truly a relief. We did not need to add to our list of problems. He suggested another internal ultra sound, which again he found to be normal. After our three-hour ordeal with "Dr. Personality," he concluded with some lab specimens needed to be obtained from both your daddy and me. No one had previously suggested your daddy was a factor in this, so we were glad to include him in the process. My blood work came back normal and we would have to wait until the next day for your daddy's results.

I went to work the next evening on night shift and asked a clerk if she could check the computer for your daddy's lab results. She was more than willing, and I sat anxiously as the computer changed screens and prepared to flash the results before me. You see, I never worried over this part of our testing because I had so many problems of my own. I knew that this was just a routine check. He couldn't be a factor in this. But to my horror, your daddy had a problem, too. In fact, he had a very serious problem for our future. My eyes raced over the screen a hundred times, reading and re-reading the results. *This must be wrong*, I thought. There it was in front of me in black and white, but I couldn't accept it. Your daddy was clinically sterile.

After it rolled over me like a bulldozer, I had mixed feelings that ranged from "Woe is me" to "When God does a miracle, He sure makes it look impossible first!" Now if that isn't being double-minded, I don't know what is.

That morning, when your daddy came to pick me up from work, I couldn't say anything to him. It felt like a terrible tragedy had occurred and I could not bring myself to tell him the dooming news. How do you tell your husband that he is sterile? Especially when neither of us suspected it was a problem in the first place. We went to bed, but I couldn't sleep. Things had gone from worse to impossible. I cried for a while and then denial set in again. I thought that maybe I had read it wrong. I jumped out of bed to call Dr. T.'s nurse, who confirmed my fears. She said that there would now be no need to keep my impending appointment and not to take this month's cycle of fertility drugs. Simply no need. Instead, we were given a six-week "break" that we did not ask for, to wait and get another analysis done.

I was crushed. The fact that we had to do nothing for six weeks was even harder to cope with. Depression started within me, accompanied by an "I-don't-care" attitude. I cried a lot and slept little. The insomnia seemed endless. During the day being motivated to get routine things accomplished felt impossible. I was tired all of the time. The house was getting filthy and the dirtier it got, the more depressed I became. I still could not get myself to do anything about the vicious cycle I was in. Along with all of that came large amounts of guilt (which just feeds depression). I knew that your daddy was carrying the biggest part of the load. I felt like I was so undeserving to have someone as tolerant as him. He was so undeserving to be stuck with someone as weak as me. It has been very trying.

While we wait to be retested, we have been researching the adoption avenue much closer. Rev. Null opened our hearts to it in May and I thought it would be the "easy way out" of our fertility problems. How I was wrong. The expense is astronomical! Most of the large agencies are money hungry, but can "produce" children within a reasonable amount of time—almost too reasonable. The smaller agencies seem to have the children's best interest at heart and are less expensive, but they could take years to find us a match and would still cost us thousands of non-refundable dollars. It's kind of a lose-lose situation. I feel so victimized by these people because they prey on our infertility. They know there are couples that can't have children, but desperately yearn for a child. They know that most couples will go to any length for a chance to become parents. This has been very traumatizing to me. I just can't seem to find an appropriate outlet.

A social worker from the hospital referred me to a nearby agency. I called them and set up an appointment to get further information from them. This was one of the "less money, more wait" agencies. To my dismay, the representative decided that she would like to meet at our home because she had some meetings out of the office that day. I was in a panic! The house was a wreck and even though this was not an "official" visit, I knew the change in plans was so they could check us out. I called a couple of ladies from the church to help me spring clean. I worked that day so they started before I got home. I joined in as soon as I got through the door and changed my clothes. It took twelve hours to get this place into shape! We scrubbed with toothbrushes and investigated every nook and cranny with some sort of cleaning supply. At last the house was back in order and immaculate. Everything sparkled.

The next day came, and I received another phone call. The agency representative wanted to come at an even earlier time to accommodate her schedule. I confidently agreed and then made another mad dash through the house trying to get everything in its place. I was a little frightened. The voice I had spoken to on the phone was very professional. I told your daddy that she would probably arrive in a business suit and a BMW. Instead, we spotted a gray Grand Am driving up to our home carrying a petite Italian lady with a gentle wave and a large smile. We shook hands and invited her in as we made our introductions. She was clad in sandals, shorts, and a knit tank top. She was very non-threatening. I felt relief pour over me as we indulged in light conversation woven with information about the adoption agency. She made several comments on our "beautiful home," which also gave me comfort. We passed the unofficial test.

During her three-hour visit, we talked about many options and decisions we would have to make regarding adoption. We also learned of the insurmountable amount of procedures and paper work we would have to be processed through just to be approved and placed on an active list. That alone could take up to three months! By the time we said goodbye we had made a new friend who wanted to work with us through our home study, if we choose this route. My head spun with all of this new information.

That evening, I sifted through the packets she brought us. There were many heartbreaking stories of international adoption situations along with references and advertisements of larger agencies. On top of everything else, there was the list of service fees. I felt so helpless and angry by that point that I wanted to light a match to the whole thing and just say forget it!

I know I am not ready to start this process yet. I feel like I have been tapped dry already. I need to rebuild the resources within me before starting a new challenge like this. I do know that if you are to come to us by adoption that God will make a way for you to get to us.

As it stands right now, we will repeat the analysis in about two and a half weeks. Those results will then determine what steps we take next, if any. If Dr. T. feels we have a chance with fertility treatments, we will try with every ounce of strength we have. If he feels we have little or no chance, we will try to prepare for an adoption plan. The nurse has informed us of some very high tech procedures that we can try to help us conceive, but they are very costly (around twenty thousand dollars) and may not even be effective for us.

As I muddle through this I still pray for a miracle, one I know down deep that I will get. I know God has to be more than disappointed in me for my wavering faith. I don't even know if I could call it wavering faith. I think it may be more of impatience and one huge pity party for myself. I am ashamed to say that through all of my depression and discouragement this month I have lost sight of you. I must keep my positive thoughts focused on you and why we are doing all of the crazy things that we are doing. I just want to be normal like everyone else. This is something that is just supposed to happen.

Another irony I have faced this month was that a friend unexpectedly became pregnant. Her husband had a vasectomy and they were shocked. She spent the whole week in tears because they already have five kids. Her husband was very upset with her as if it were her fault. Isn't it amazing how I cry myself to sleep at night because I can't have children, while she cries herself to sleep because she has too many? It is an unfair world that we live in.

Well, my love, I have poured out all that I can for the present time. I must say that this has been quite therapeutic for me. I skipped church tonight because I couldn't deal with having to wear my fake smile and "my-life-is-great" look again. I think that this has really helped, though. I love you and I am still impatiently waiting to wake up from this nightmare. I keep thinking about how special you must be for heaven not to want to give you up quite so easily! You must be quite a treasure.

With all my love,
Mommy

July 25, 1998

To my angel baby,

My dear angel, we have hit bottom. It has been a long journey and we have now reached the end of our road. I believe it was the 14th of the month that your daddy had his repeat analysis done. It was even worse than the first one—if that could be possible! I just couldn't accept that. We prayed, we had hoped for the best, even for just a slight improvement, but it became worse instead.

After obtaining the results, I called Dr. T.'s nurse. She gently handed me the death sentence—the death sentence of my dream. My heart plummeted as these words, "There is nothing else we can do. I am sorry, Mrs. Donham," pierced through the telephone receiver directly to my tattered heart. I helplessly sobbed as I hung up the phone. She had reminded me of our option to try that high-tech procedure, but it is just too costly and so new that they are not sure if there would be long-term effects on the children conceived by it. So our choice became no child or one that could be genetically mutilated.

I have been bitter in my spirit. I can't handle this anymore! It has become a burden too heavy to bear. I have given up, sweet baby. I have no option for a biological child, and affording and obtaining a child by adoption is just mind-boggling. At this time I don't know if I will ever be able to go through with that whole process. I just can't. So, my angel baby, you will live on in my heart and in my wishes, but I guess I must wait until I get to heaven to hold you in my arms. That is devastating to me, but I am helpless. I have no control.

This is one obstacle that will continue to battle me—the

helplessness. Every one assumes this is something I can control and that I just choose not to have a child. That angers me greatly! I can't help it! It often brings me to tears. God has control of this—not me. I am finished with this. People around me continue to get pregnant while I remain childless. It's so painful. I quit!

I have handed my shattered pieces over to God. If He wants me to have you, He will have to give me the miracle in His own timing. I am so tired of begging. So if you are supposed to be, let it be done. If not, I pray that He helps me with this throbbing in my heart for you so that I can live the rest of my life without this constant turmoil and agony. I am so sorry that I let you down. I love you, my sweet desire. You will always be my angel baby.

I'll see you in heaven,

Mommy

October 15, 1998

To my sweet angel baby,

I have been in utter despair since I wrote you last. Life has lost meaning. I was fine for a few weeks and thought nothing of this desire. One day while working in the nursery at the hospital, it all came flooding back with tidal waves of hurt and pain washing over me.

I looked at all of the precious newborns that surrounded me as thoughts of their mother's pregnancies filled my mind. I wondered how each of them celebrated and prepared for their new arrivals. How happy they must have been to have these sweet infants in their lives. I watched as a new father looked proudly over his crying newborn son with tears filling his eyes. That's when it hit me. We wouldn't be able to experience any of these treasures of life. I desperately attempted to choke my tears back for fear that someone would notice my distress.

There were a few infants that I am sure didn't receive the reception they deserved. They were probably unplanned or one of a string of many. One was being given to a couple to adopt. How my arms ached. I held, fed and cared for infants all day, yet my arms felt empty. I felt isolated in a room crammed with medical staff, students and babies. I felt myself sinking into anguish again. Since that day I have jumped back on the emotional roller coaster, with all of its day-to-day ups and downs.

As I told you before, I have given up. Yet even in my despondency, I still yearn for you. I can't understand why I have been withheld from this awesome privilege. I have prayed, cried and had all the faith I could possibly have, with only dashed hopes and dreams as a result.

I feel so incompetent. I just can't stand this! I have sought after God and done all I know to do. What now? Every option has been exhausted and my only hope, God, just doesn't seem to care. I feel like He won't respond to me or my prayers.

I am now mourning your loss and what never came to be. Every month when I start a new cycle I wish for my insides to just shrivel up and fall out. If they are not going to work and provide the life they were made to hold—what is the use? It just creates more false hopes that lower me deeper into my depression. At least then there would be no chance left, and I could permanently grieve your loss. Instead, I have month after month of hope and loss.

I felt like something different was occurring in my life. It happened so fast and miraculously that I expected you to come closely after. In one week we received our family-sized car, your daddy got a promotion, and I got the job that I have been praying for. My new job permitted me to go part-time. This will allow me to be a stay-at-home mommy someday. After we were blessed to this extent, I naturally thought that you would just follow. When you didn't, I was crushed. The depression is back and worse than ever. It is so hard to deal with it all. I am now at work learning my new job, but I still can't get you out of my thoughts.

Today, my mind drifts back to July when I was upset by the news that your daddy's counts were worse. My friend, Christy, came over to me in church and prayed with me. She said that God spoke to her heart and she felt that within three months time God would give me my answer, or at least the direction He would take me in. Well, this Saturday (October17th) is the deadline. My cycle is due to start and I am getting all of the physical signs that it will start. I have been so hopeful that this would be it. Now it is looking like I am getting my answer, that it isn't God's plan for me to give birth.

I must confess that with each passing day I do have a glimmer of hope welling up inside of me. I am trying to smother those feelings because I think that I am setting myself up for another heartbreak. I just hate it! I don't know what I am supposed to do without you. I don't understand why God would promise you to me, but not allow you to come.

I am now subjected to those who can produce babies left and right, but not even want them. It is so unimaginable to me. I just can't stand the irony here. I am so sorry I am not good enough for you to come to me. I am so very sorry.

In the midst of the chaos that has attacked my mind and emotions, I face another devastating circumstance. I want to tell you about a very special person, your Great-grandpa Musick. I was hoping you would come to us before any of your great-grandparents left here, but it looks like your Great-grandpa Musick will be coming your way anytime now. We almost lost him last week and now the doctors say he only has two or three months with us. Grandpa's life is slipping away hastily. Even though he has lived a full life, it still feels premature for him to be going anywhere.

My memory entertains me with happy thoughts of me as a child tipping on Grandpa's heels under a blue sky and warm sun. We would walk in his lush garden picking peas and beans. We would find a good spot on the ground to have one of our simple talks and eat raw peas as the warm summer breeze embraced us. Grandpa would help me up with his strong, work-worn hand as I dusted the dirt off, wondering what adventure Grandpa and I could embark on next.

The most touching thing Grandpa ever did for me is twofold. First, he cried at my wedding. Your daddy sang a song to me during the ceremony. Afterward, we turned to face our family and friends again. My eyes fell to the front of the church where my family sat and I saw Grandpa wiping the tears from his eyes. No doubt his thoughts turned back to our days in the garden, too. Then at our reception came an even sweeter and unexpected gift from Grandpa. As everyone was getting lost in their food and conversation, Grandpa quietly approached the bridal table. He didn't say a word; he just opened his mouth and began to sing, "May God grant you many years" first in Slovak, then in English. It was such a precious moment between us. Only those who were sitting close had the privilege of witnessing

Grandpa expressing his love to us in a very touching way.

We also had a special moment in the hospital together. As he lay ill in the hospital bed feeling defeated by his cancer, I reached over and grabbed hold of his once strong hand. His feeble grip became firm in mine as I tried to encourage him with thoughts of heaven and what it will be like for him to experience. I gave him every descriptive detail about heaven that I could remember from my years in church. He lay with his head resting on a pillow and his eyes shut. I could see the worry in his expression, knowing his time was now short. I announced to Grandpa that I needed a favor. I told him that I had been trying for a very long time to get my angel baby here before any of my grandparents left me. And right now, it seemed everyone was trying to be quite stubborn. My baby wouldn't come, and Grandpa kept trying to leave! It was putting me in a real difficult spot, I teased. So I asked him for the favor. I told him that when he got to heaven, he needed to find you and send you to me. I asked if he would mind doing that for me. He opened his eyes for just a moment, broke out into a wide smile, and patted my hand. As if being sent on a mission, he confidently told me he would do that for me. It seemed to give Grandpa a sense of purpose and me a sense of hope.

Give him lots of love and care when he gets to heaven. It will be so new to him. Tell him how much I love and miss him. I am going to hang onto him for as long as I can, though.

I hope that one day I will be able to meet you in heaven. Then I will hold you close and have you for eternity. I guess, my angel baby, you will remain just that—an angel. I love you and I will see you in heaven.

With all of my love,

Mommy

October 21, 1998

My dear angel baby,

I grieve heavily for you today. I sit here at work with my head in my hands not knowing how I am going to get through this day. So much has come upon me that it magnifies my life without you.

Someday I will tell you all about your cousin, baby Hope. She is currently thirteen months old. Her mommy is ill and doesn't really want to care for her like she should. She has been staying with us a good bit for the last month. There has been talk of your daddy and me adopting baby Hope. Again, I have had such mixed emotions as before, and this time I am afraid she will never truly be mine. The adoption situation would be much different in this case because her birth parents would probably always be within arm's reach. I don't know if that would give us the freedom we would need to be her parents. She is so sweet, though. She has an innocently precious face with large, round hazel eyes. Her smile melts my heart. There is a certain sadness about her, though. Probably because she has never really been settled in one home for any great length of time.

It seems like every time I let my guard down and open my heart up, it just gets trampled upon. I am so weary with this. Last week, I decided that this was it. If we got the word, I would do all in my power to adopt Hope. With her staying so often, I was enjoying the fantasy of being her mother and having a child in our home. That was until last Sunday. Her birth mom showed up at church (which was a rare occasion) long enough to whisk Hope into her arms as Hope innocently smiled with excitement. None of this meant that she was ready to be the mother Hope needed and longed for. It was simply to prove a point: "I can waltz in any time I want and be recognized as her mother." My insides went to pieces, what was left of them, that is.

Then I started with the questions again. Is this the way it would be her whole life with us? Would she ever love us like she loves her biological parents? Would this be the right thing to pursue—is it God's will? I just didn't know if I could deal with the reality of the answers to those questions. Everywhere we go I hear "Oh, that's P— 's baby, she looks so much like P—." People may not realize it, but I don't need reminded of who gave birth to Hope. They always fail to recognize who is caring for Hope. It certainly is not P—.

As much as I love baby Hope and want to keep her, I wish that you were here too. It would make it so much easier because I wouldn't feel like such a failure. I then could love her unconditionally because those remarks would be painless. It's not going to happen that way, though, is it?

On top of it all, I have to deal with everyone else's emotional lows when I don't even feel strong enough for myself. I am helping with the care of your Great-grandpa Musick. It is so hard seeing him ill. I just never imagined that things would ever turn this way regarding his health. He was always such a strong person. It is pitiful seeing him overcome by cancer. I can't stand it! I am such an emotional basket case that I don't even want to be around myself!

I had such a stressful day yesterday. Things just kept piling and piling against me. I felt I was doing a good job handling the pressure, although I could feel it getting harder. Finally, about 9:30 p.m., I decided that I would try to escape the insanity by going to bed. That didn't help. I just tossed until I heard the phone ring. Trouble! I could sense it. I sprung out of bed and bolted to the living room in time to see your daddy's worried expression. Then I heard him give a sorrowful, "Oh no." I grabbed for the caller ID to find his parents' number listed. I asked, "What? What?" My heart pounded as a million thoughts of tragedy raced through my frantic mind.

He covered the phone receiver and said, "It's Deanna, apparently she is having a miscarriage, and she is about two months and … " I threw up my hand and said I didn't want to know as I burst into tears and fled to my bedroom again. It felt so traumatic. Just one more bad thing to squeeze itself into the day as a precious life had been lost. I knew Deanna seemed different, never dreaming she was pregnant. One more life had been given, and then abruptly taken. I got so angry with God. I just couldn't take it! I cried myself to sleep in the midst of my emotions whirling around inside me, tormenting any last morsels of solace I may have had.

I woke this morning with the same sadness hanging over me. What an oppression. I want to run away, but I am sure it will follow me. I don't have time for these feelings. There are so many other areas in my life that need attention right now. I need a way out of this turmoil, but what? I have been taught that the answer should be God. But every time I call upon Him, He seems to turn a deaf ear.

Your daddy does not seem to understand where I am in this. I think he just doesn't get it, or he is so optimistic that he feels things are just fine. I know he is definitely not tuned in to the same channel as me. That makes things all the more painful.

I am absolutely alone in this nightmare. Friends try to give advice and help, but they still don't quite understand. I don't think anyone except women who have agonized with infertility can truly acknowledge the pain of it.

I turn to pen and paper to empty my soul to you, dear baby. It provides me some relief, but not a cure. Hopefully, this will help me manage through my day. I am thankful my back is to my coworkers in the office because tears are sliding down my face uncontrollably. It is going to be a hard day in all of this darkness.

I love you,
Mommy

October 27, 1998

My dear angel baby,

Not a whole lot is different today. My emotions still rage as they scrape bottom. I feel I am able to breathe today. I still feel the pain of everything and can be reduced to tears within a heartbeat.

I know I have said that I had given up, but I find myself still addicted to you. Now I make one last dismal attempt at the pursuit of my dream. We have learned of another option that we can try. It is a surgical procedure that could possibly restore your daddy's fertility. We scheduled an appointment for November 3rd to arrange for surgery. I am hoping and praying that the surgery will be around Thanksgiving. Then maybe we could resume fertility treatments in December. What a Christmas present that would be! Oh, how I hoped and prayed that you would be here by this Christmas, or at least that I'd be pregnant for you.

I am sure that the holidays are going to be a bit distressing. I had set goals in faith and once again they have gone unmet. I usually look forward to the holidays, but this year I feel like I am going to ruin them for myself. I am scared because I don't want to make myself or anyone else around me miserable.

It is funny how I feel numb, yet experience so much pain. Why won't you come to us, dear baby? I had such wonderful plans for our lives. They have come to a sudden halt. What now? Every time I gather enough strength to pick up and start again, I am knocked back and stopped in my tracks. How do I get a hold on this thing? Will I ever gain control? We want you so desperately, sweet baby. What does God have planned for us? Does He really hear our prayers and see our tears? Will God ever replace this sadness with joy? I want to be happy again. I can't remember what that is like anymore.

I am not so naive to think that your arrival will fix everything in our lives. I do know the immense joy you would bring to us and all of our family. It would renew my faith and restore my hopes and dreams just knowing that miracles do happen. Will you ever come to us, or am I entangled in this tug-of-war for no reason at all? Please come to us, precious child. We love you so much already. Please come.

Longing as I wait,

Mommy

October 30, 1998

To my sweet angel baby,

Well, my dear child, I have made the appointment for your father and surgery looks likely for the week of Thanksgiving as we had hoped. Could it be our dreams are becoming reality? Oh, how thankful I will be to have this over with. Prayerfully, you will be coming soon after this surgical intervention is complete.

Just when I have gained the will to place my focus on you again, change comes about. I feel so fragile that my emotions are about to shatter. Last evening, I spoke with your Grammy. P— had called and once again made mention of us adopting Hope. I am so confused. How am I supposed to feel? Every time I allow myself to become happy or excited, things always turn in the other direction, leaving me to crumble into useless little pieces.

We just started thinking of you again and once more the tables turn. I don't want to delay your arrival, but I don't want to deny Hope the love, attention and good home that she needs and deserves. We honestly want to give her that, but I am also yearning deeply for you, my angel baby. You're the greatest desire I have ever had and nothing but you will quench that thirst. You are not to be replaced. Hope could never replace you, nor could you ever replace Hope.

This has been a separate painful situation in itself that I have not written much about because my focal point has always been you— the reason for these letters. Please know, dear child, if all works out you may have a big sister waiting on you when you come!

Anxiously anticipating you,

Mommy

November 10, 1998

To my sweet angel,

So much has happened once again since I wrote last. On October 30th, P— called and asked that we start the paperwork to adopt our precious little Hope. Fear and excitement surged through me simultaneously! I kept thinking that the whirlwind has just begun.

By the end of last week she had already changed her mind four times! That ended with her finally keeping Hope. I was in anguish, especially after learning that she took her just to drop her off to another sitter. That dear child was in four homes in one short week!

We did keep our appointment with the urologist and scheduled surgery for November 23rd. That is the Monday of Thanksgiving week. We at least have that to rely upon.

To add to all of this chaos, things fell apart once again in Hope's home and it looks like she is coming back to us. Only God knows for how long.

Dear angel baby, how I wish you were here with us. It just seems like things would be a little better for having you with us. We still pray for you to come. I am becoming cautiously hopeful that this procedure your daddy is about to have will be our answer for you. Like I said before, you might very well have a big sister waiting on you. You will love her, precious baby. Have a wonderful day in heaven.

With increasing faith,
Mommy

January 15, 1999

To my precious angel,

I have so much to tell you about since I wrote last. Let me back up to November 23rd, your daddy's surgery. I think we were both nervous, but we made it through that day as the urologist made the necessary repair. We were prayerfully thinking of you while we went through this procedure. All went well except your daddy had a reaction to the anesthesia. They gave him too much. But God kept His hand upon him and he recovered well. I don't think he even took a pain pill! The disappointing part is that we won't know if the surgery worked until February 4th. We have to wait 72 days after surgery to repeat his counts. This should give us an accurate reading.

It was upsetting to have another delay. Hopefully it will be worth it, though. We only have a two and a half-month time frame to ensure your arrival by the end of 1999. It doesn't look optimistic. Oh please, dear God, hear our prayers! Oh well, we are only a couple of weeks away now. But again, your daddy thankfully recovered well.

To our great sadness and loss, your Great-grandpa Musick passed away and went to heaven. Has he found you yet? What do you think of him? Please give him all of my love and tell him how much I miss him. I sent him on a mission to find you, so I couldn't help but to have a sense of joy buried under the grief when he passed. I would like to think he is looking after you now and cuddling you in heaven until your time comes to be with us.

The morning he passed away your daddy and I had similar dreams at the same time. It was a bit eerie, but exciting as well. It was almost prophetic. Your daddy dreamed he was on a long dark road with a bright light in the distance. He said he could feel a light breeze blowing against him. He felt very happy and joyful. He was dancing and skipping toward the bright light. He could see someone in the distance doing the same thing behind him. Then he realized it was Grandpa Musick! At that moment, they were lifted up at a great speed through the atmosphere, until they reached a courtroom-type place in heaven. His Aunt Barbara was there beside of him in the stands.

Your daddy started to fade out of the dream and as he did Barbara asked him, "Aren't you going to take your baby, Jody?"

Then Grandpa Musick said, "Take your son." Then he woke up. At the same time, I was dreaming, too.

I dreamed I was at someone's house and I remember being in a small living room with a Christmas tree in the left-hand corner. Beside that tree was an open doorway with a step up into the kitchen. On that step lay a huge beautiful baby boy, the same one that I had seen many times over in dreams past. I remember feeling confused and excited at the same time, trying to figure out whose baby this was. *Is it mine*? I thought I as I struggled for an answer.

Your daddy's Aunt Barbara came into the room and I said, "Is he mine?"

She said, "Yes!" Like, of course he is yours, silly!

"Pick up your baby, Dorothy," Barbara exclaimed. I grabbed him up into my arms as tears poured. I held him so close; I didn't want to let him go. I rubbed his soft being in between squeezes of love. I took in that wonderful "baby smell" he was fragranced with. I will never forget the beautiful features he had as long as I live. Enormously round cheeks, soft tender skin that was milky in color, and dark blond hair that stood on end a little. He was so heavy! My arms were finally full and overflowing! Then I woke up with tears still running over my face. I desperately wanted to go back to him. My empty arms throbbed to hold him again.

I hope and pray these dreams are prophetic of your arrival. They just made me hunger even more for you! I think these dreams have been the most positive thing to occur as far as you're concerned.

During my journey through infertility I found out that a good friend of mine had secretly been fighting the same battle. We became close and shared our "war stories" and compared "battle scars." We tried everything together. When I would hear of something new to try, I would inform her and vice-versa. It didn't matter how crazy or radical the idea; anything was worth a try at least once! From pink rose quartz to eating ears of fresh corn daily, our crazy list could go on forever. We never wanted to miss an opportunity no matter how extreme. She was so sensitive about the longing for her child that I prayed God would bless her first. I literally didn't think she could handle it if I became pregnant before her. I can't believe I am saying this, but I believe I was the stronger of the two of us. That's saying a lot for how she felt!

At the end of October, we went to your Aunt Shelly and Uncle Greg's church. We were prayed for by their congregation in hopes God would hear their prayers and we would conceive our babies. They have had approximately ten couples to have the same longing, receive prayer, and then be blessed. We figured it couldn't hurt us to try either. So there we stood hand in hand at the front of the church as your daddy's brother-in-law held a service around our petitions. The church bestowed their love upon us in a faith-filled prayer. God had to hear them in all of their humbleness and humility. We just knew He had to hear their prayers.

Just a few weeks later, Heather found out she was pregnant! We were ecstatic. God had honored us! I was so happy for them, but I do admit to feeling twinges of jealousy as I questioned God when my turn would be. I also felt a lot more alone. I lost my companion in this struggle. Thankfully I lost her. Her first ultra sound confirmed what I was suspecting—twins! She had been doubly blessed. We joked with them and asked if they had a boy and a girl, which would they want to keep?

Then that inevitable Sunday morning came that I had tried very hard to prepare myself for. I knew there would be an announcement to the church that Heather and Gary were now expecting twins. It was wonderful news and they deserved to be congratulated, but I knew that deep down inside, it was going to hurt because I was once again alone in my struggle, and still empty-handed. I sat in my pew with butterflies in my stomach, praying I could hold myself together when something was said. I didn't want to make a scene or take away from this very special occasion. As your Pap-pap Donham started making his announcements from the pulpit, I drew a deep breath in. Christy, who was sitting with me, asked if I was going to be OK. Patting my hand, she knew the awkward position I was in as I fought back the tears. I shook my head yes as the announcement blared through the sound system. When the church applauded and gave their congratulations, I turned my head, biting my quivering lips as my tears that I attempted to imprison escaped me. I struggled to capture those feelings and bury them again. Finally succeeding, I wiped the tears away and lifted my head.

I had done fine with the news until Christmas. I knew Christmas would be tough anyway. It was getting harder year by year. I bought Heather a picture I had been looking at for years to place in my future nursery. It is a beautiful picture of a mother lovingly holding her infant close. It is inscribed, "For this child I have prayed." I was anxious to give it to her, knowing the special meaning it would have. But as I was wrapping it, I broke down. I lost it. I couldn't bear wrapping for her what I thought would be mine for Christmas. I didn't want to feel that way, but I couldn't help it. Your daddy draped his arms around me and held me as I continued to weep. After I regained a little strength, I continued on. I wrapped and sobbed with your daddy until I had a beautiful tear-stained gold package.

Christmas was also especially hard without Grandpa Musick and you. I barely made it through. I knew it wouldn't be quite as bad with my side of the family, but on your daddy's side there were a few new babies and it was bound to be hard. We had Hope with us, it was our first Christmas together. As soon as we arrived everyone oohed and aahed over Hope. A well-meaning person commented, "You look almost normal with her!" I was completely mortified. I knew I felt abnormal, but no one had informed me that you had to give birth to a child to look like a "normal" mother. I didn't even have my coat off and I already had my heart stomped on.

The day wore on with more encounters that challenged my impersonation of being a mother and the infertility I struggled with. I was very proud that I kept a stiff upper lip until we got into the car. I buried my head in my lap and cried all of the way home. That was my Christmas memory for 1998.

New Years has been quite emotional, too. The chance of me having a child in the 20th century isn't likely. We have until March to conceive and I am not very optimistic. I try not to think about it because it is so depressing. We have nothing to do but wait, pray and watch the time go by without you.

We do have Hope, but she is another story. We hired a lawyer, but right now things are on shaky ground. I can't seem to let myself get excited about anything or depend on anyone any more. It is all too back and forth. We are just holding on and waiting.

On February 4th, your daddy is having his post-surgical count done. I have had a sick gut feeling about it. I am afraid, dear baby. I have let my faith dwindle and seep out of me. I pray I am wrong. I want you so bad, sweet angel.

Carefully watching for you,

Mommy

February 11, 1999

Dear angel baby,

We have lost, sweet child. It looks like we will not hold you in this millennium. My heart has been crushed. On February 4th, we received the long awaited post-surgical values. It seems that they are even worse than before surgery. This was not supposed to happen! I totally lost my mind with the news. Our chances of ever conceiving are impossible now. Even the doctors are dumbfounded with the bewildering results.

I have cried for days on end. I can't get this out of my heart. I feel the loss to the depths of my soul. I am so upset with God because I have nowhere else to turn. It feels like He has abandoned me in this hellish nightmare. Why am I being punished so harshly? I don't understand anymore. The pain and confusion are more than I can bear, dear child.

After we received the results we immediately started questioning why this was happening to us. Your daddy implied that maybe I didn't have enough faith, and that is why things were not working out. I was already living on the brink of insanity and that statement plunged me over the edge.

We said some bitter words back and forth until I found myself needing to escape the heated moment. I turned and ran into the bathroom. As I locked the door behind me, I felt as if someone delivered a tremendous blow to my soul with a sledgehammer. The pain was so deep and intense I wailed in agony. I collapsed and curled up into a ball on the floor. I held my legs tightly against my chest, hoping I could fold myself inside out and just disappear. Between sobs I started screaming out at God at the top of my lungs, "Take the pain away. Take away my desire! If you are not going to give me my baby, take away the desire. I don't want it anymore! This hurts so bad, please take away the pain!" My body shook and quivered as the cries ripped away from my agonizing soul. The sheer brutality of the pain scared me. At that moment, I felt like I separated from myself and was now watching the horrific scene from a distance. I was sure I was having a nervous breakdown and I didn't think I would come out of that room on my own.

This went on for close to two hours. As the uncontrollable sobs continued, the part of me on the floor wanted to hate God for His abandonment, while the part of me that watched felt His presence fill that room. It was then that my spirit started to groan in intercession out of the limp body slumped on the cold floor. I felt God's hand reaching toward me to caress and hold me, like a father would console a child after getting hurt. I believe He was hurting with me and shed tears as He "held" me in my despair.

After I allowed myself to acknowledge His presence with me, I slowly regained composure and finally answered your daddy's frantic calls for me at the bathroom door. I weakly got up and the room spun around me. I felt as if my life source had been tapped and drained. I fumbled to the door and fell into your daddy's arms where I cried some more while we talked through our pain.

That was the most terrifying, dark moment of my life. I never want to sink that low again. When I even revisit that time in my mind, I shudder. I still don't know what would have happened to me if God had not intervened.

I am now considering counseling. I just don't know how else to pick up the shattered pieces from my tragic ordeal. I feel like I have known nothing but heartache and devastation.

We are still struggling to keep Hope. The adoption papers are ready, but they won't sign them. That has been it's own horrendous ordeal. I have packed and unpacked baby Hope's tattered bags so many times, I am not sure if she is coming or going. I wonder if God will allow Hope to leave us too, despite all of the prayers we have prayed on her behalf.

I just need a way out of this suffering, sweet baby. I have never wanted anything more in my life than you. Things are in an impossible position now, but deep down inside I know I will always be saying a prayer for you to come to me. I will desire you for eternity, sweet angel. I know now I will have to wait until I get to heaven to hold you. Then I will never let you go.

Forever in my dreams,

Mommy

October 1, 1999

Dearest Angel,

After that fateful turning point in February, numbness overshadowed my pain. Day by day I grew stronger, but my heart grew harder. I had absolutely no faith that I would ever give birth to you. I was able to breathe again, but I still didn't feel alive. I didn't want to be involved with church, work, or anything else that used to hold importance to me. I was totally desensitized to my surroundings. I did what I had to, just to get by. I felt like I was living in a dreamlike state of mind as I dragged myself through my days, almost aimlessly. I couldn't concentrate on anything. I felt like life had lost its purpose.

We struggled to keep Hope in our lives. Days after the last entry in my journal, God moved in a powerful way. The birth mother signed the first set of adoption papers relinquishing all rights to Hope on February 23, 1999. The birth father was out of town and unable to sign his set of documents. For the first time relief entered my mind. God was giving us a child. We met with our friend Kelly, and drove to Pittsburgh to celebrate at the Olive Garden. It felt so good to smile again.

The celebration didn't last long. The birth mother had manipulated the birth father into not signing his set of adoption papers, tying up the whole process and putting agonizing delays on the adoption finalization. We battled with these people as we tried to reason with them and encourage them to finish what they had started. Many prayers went up from our church, family and friends. After many tears and distressing phone calls, our burden was relieved.

Several months had passed before the second set of adoption papers was signed. Hope was finally going to be ours.

On Mother's Day, May 9, 1999, we had little Hope dedicated to the Lord. It was a bittersweet occasion for me. I was so thankful that the Lord had blessed us with her and brought us through the ordeal of having the papers signed, but I still had that yearning down deep for you, too.

I cuddled Hope on my lap at her dedication with tears trickling down my face as my dad spoke. He reminded us that God could still bless us with another child and that he felt that He would. This was so painful to hear because it stirred those old feelings back up. It also made me feel like a failure, not being strong enough to be happy for my darling Hope. I still allowed my emotions to be twisted and contorted by my addiction of wanting you. I also was dealing with the excruciating realization of Mother's Day. I was sitting on a pew "pretending" to be a mother, when in fact the adoption had not been finalized, and I still did not have you here.

We went on to have a beautiful service for Hope. Your daddy sang a song to our little girl that I wrote for her. It summed up the whole event for us:

"Hope's Song"

Verse 1—We planned our lives so perfect. We made our wishes and dreamed our dreams. The future looked so bright, but it was not what it seemed. As disappointments came our way we cried, "God, why is life unfair?" He spoke, "Child be still and you will know I care. Yes, I see the path your walking, know that I do have a plan. As I guide you to the open door—toward the gift I have in store..." (Chorus)

Chorus—You are a gift of mercy. You are a gift from up above. God looked down upon our sorrow and replaced it with your love. You are a gift of mercy. You are our destiny. We're so blessed by you, angel. You made us a family.

Verse 2—You're not flesh of my flesh. Yet still precious, child of mine. Not by our creation. You're our child by God's design. Yes, we struggled deep within with what we thought should be. Then God gave us you, and taught us what makes "family." We never knew how love could mend a broken heart. We've learned so much from you and this is just the start! (Repeat chorus)

Verse 3—Lord, we want to thank you for giving abundantly. What you've given us in love, we give back humbly. She's a gift so undeserved, yet You still cared for us. We'll raise her for Your glory and in You we'll always trust. We pray for Your wisdom as we teach her all of Your ways. We'll tell her how You brought her to us, and this is what we'll say... (Repeat chorus)

God continued to do a work in our hearts as we adjusted to our new family and fell deeper in love with Hope as each new day passed.

On June 19th, 1999, Grammy and Aunt Kathy had a baby shower for Hope and me. That was something I thought I would never have the honor to experience. It was very odd to have a trim-bellied mother and the guest of honor present to unwrap her gifts. It was quite a happy occasion, but I still felt awkward. I wondered when someone would reveal the truth of my masquerade. It felt like at any given moment, the whole scam would crumble and there I would be— childless again and humiliated for pretending to be something I was not. These feelings of inadequacy would take a long time to resolve.

Finally, the long awaited day arrived. On July 6, 1999, Hope's adoption finalization took place. None of our family was permitted to attend, because this was a closed adoption. It was just our lawyer, a stenographer, the judge, and us. It was a very intimidating scene as we sat quietly in this cavernous courtroom, trying to keep our squirming 22-month old entertained and respectful. It eased our minds to learn that the judge who presided over our case had adopted his children also. We knew that he would be quite understanding of our feelings on this special day.

Our lawyer presented our case and documents to the judge as we juggled Hope quietly between us. Then the judge had several questions to ask us and we seemed to stutter back the answers. He kindly asked if we had anything to say for the court's record and each of us spoke of the gratitude we had in our hearts for this opportunity with Hope and of how we were smitten with this precious little girl. He smiled a smile of having been there himself and informed us that this was the great part of his job. Daily he dealt with murder trials and other crimes, but today he got to see a beautiful child placed in a wonderful home, with two adoring parents.

Our lawyer had previously warned us not to get our hope up because the judge would typically not sign the papers at the hearing. It would probably take several weeks. But to our astonishment, he asked that the papers be turned over to him, and he signed them before us! Hope was now legally our little girl—Hope Alexandra Donham, and nothing could change that! We were finally parents. After that surprising gesture, the judge did something else quite unexpected. He stepped down off of his bench and came down to our seats to shake our hands and congratulate us. He scooped little Hope into his arms and hugged her as she delicately pointed out the characters in a book she was playing with. We all giggled as she baby-talked their names in her quaint little voice.

We left the courtroom hugging and thanking our lawyer as we rushed home to tell our family of the day's details. We could rest our hearts and minds now. This ordeal had come to an end. You now have a sister, precious baby.

Hope's adoption reminded me of the story of "The Three Trees." In the end, each of the trees got what they had wished for, just not in the way that they imagined. God had a very special plan for us. I know His ways are not our ways. But His ways are always best. And we were blessed with a beautiful little girl as a result.

On September 2nd, we planned a huge birthday party to celebrate Hope's second birthday. Over one hundred people were invited, and Hope's birth father attended. Things went smoothly as we shared this special day with all of Hope's family and friends. Not once did our parenthood collide with the birth father. We all understood and respected the new roles we now played in Hope's life.

God has done some major repair in my heart. He has given me a "spiritual epidural," as the pain of my infertility has felt anesthetized. However, I still experience breakthrough pain from time to time. Our new life with Hope gives me just that—hope. She is able to divert my attention away from most of the pain, even though I am prone to relapses.

As time goes by, I allow myself to fall deeper under Hope's spell. I am completely charmed by her character. It is not nearly as difficult to enjoy parent/child adventures with her as it was in the beginning. I am slowly able to quit comparing my "wished for life" to the one I am living. I am finally able to open my heart completely to Hope and hold her there. As Hope's love infiltrates my life, I am losing concentration on my past.

With renewed hope,

Mommy

May 10, 2000

To my precious little angel baby,

My heart is doing flip-flops! I am so ecstatic because I never believed I would ever be able to write to you again. Surprisingly, an unexpected twist of fate has necessitated another entry in my journal that I thought I had tucked away forever. I have smiled all day long! It is now near midnight and I am too euphoric to sleep. Why? Because we are finally on the brink of our miracle—You! I am still flabbergasted at this astonishing news. After four of the most painful years of my life, I am happy again!

A few weeks ago, I learned that a friend of mine became pregnant after many years of trying. I was thrilled for her. I can't even imagine the emotions that she felt upon learning her miracle had finally arrived. I believe it was sheer joy. I was at the mall shopping and happened to bump into her and her mother. I instantly threw my arms up with a huge smile on my face and headed her direction. As I congratulated her on her new pregnancy she delivered the grim news that she had actually miscarried the pregnancy a week and a half prior. I was so horrified that I had opened my big mouth without thinking! Of all people, I certainly knew better than to speak before I thought. I felt the heat radiating about my face as it flushed red. I tried desperately to keep my composure. I stuttered an apology to her and gave her my condolences. I later cried in my car all of the way home because I felt so terrible.

While I tried my best to apologize to her, we attempted to steer the uncomfortable conversation in another direction. She had asked what your daddy and I had planned, if anything, to achieve a pregnancy. I told her that we were permanently on hold due to the excessive cost of the procedure that we needed. She asked exactly what procedure we needed that was so unattainable. I told her that it was IVF/ICSI and that it would cost close to twenty thousand dollars at the clinic we were referred to. I also told her that our doctor had callously told us to try it once and if it didn't work out , "Just go raise sheep dogs instead." With a puzzled look she informed me that she had the very same procedure and it was less than half the cost! She also informed me that the procedure was done right here in West Virginia. Immediately we started swapping information and phone numbers as she encouraged me to check it out—and that I did.

The next morning at 8 a.m. sharp I was on the phone calling Dr. T.'s office. I knew little of the adventure I would encounter just trying to obtain a referral to Charleston. I couldn't even get my calls returned by his office. I was standing on the threshold of everything I had ever prayed for and I couldn't get a call back from my doctor! My nerves were frazzled, to say the least. After two and a half weeks and five phone calls, I finally got my call returned by Dr. T. himself. With little help or concern from his part, I was able to pull the information I needed from him to get things rolling. When I called Dr. Y.'s office in Charleston, I was shocked to receive an appointment so swiftly. May 10, 2000.

As we prepared for our appointment, we looked over the figures once again. It certainly would cost less than the initial twenty thousand dollars we were told we would have to pay, but somehow we still were not sure if we could afford this. We decided to keep the appointment anyway and learn what we could about the procedure and our chances. If we couldn't afford it right now, maybe we could save money and proceed with it at a later date. I was not sure if that would be a good thing because we would once again not be able to move forward.

As we set out on our two and a half-hour drive, I struggled to hold the tears back once more. All of the old feelings and thoughts of impossibilities took over my mind and once again held it captive for the trip to Charleston. I had been told no so many times in the past.

Why in the world did I think that this time it would be any different? Was I crazy? Faith and fear battled inside of my mind, each determined to rule. I fought the urge to tell your daddy to just turn the car around and go home before we surrendered ourselves to disappointment once again. I resisted that urge and we drove on.

When we finally arrived at the clinic, I wiped my red eyes dry and we nervously headed for the office. My stomach churned and my hands trembled. When we entered the cramped waiting room, I was shaking so bad that I dropped my medical records. All eyes were on me as I hurriedly fumbled through my scattered mess, trying to clean it up. I nervously shoved papers back into their disheveled file and proceeded to the registration desk. We finally managed to sign in and find a seat without making a further scene.

After a short waiting period, my name was called and we were escorted to a nursing area where my weight and vital signs were collected and recorded. We were then greeted by Dr. Y.'s nurse. She welcomed us and settled us into a cozy little conference room to watch a video about infertility and the procedures available to us. It was familiar territory for me, but I appreciated the refresher anyway. I think your daddy gained a little respect for what I would have to endure in the future as details of the procedure flashed before us.

After a brief interlude, Dr. Y. came and introduced himself as he joined us to take an extensive health history. He was a very kind gentleman with a spark of humor that made us feel at ease. After our lengthy conversation, I headed for ultrasound and your daddy was sent to the lab, as our exams would begin. Nothing new was obtained, but we did learn that we were perfect candidates for in vitro fertilization and intra cytoplasmic sperm injection.

Basically, we were told, "When you're ready, we're ready." I couldn't believe my ears.

"Could you repeat that again, please?" I stammered in shock. No impossibilities? No waiting? No new problems? I was in total disbelief! Dr. Y. continued to reassure us and moved us along for phase two.

With one hurdle out of the way, we raced toward the next. It was time to meet with their financial counselor. We were led to her office, and as she sorted through my insurance information, she said, "Your insurance should cover most of the procedure, Mrs. Donham." My mouth dropped open. I asked her if she was sure, and had her review the figures with me, which she confidently did. Once again, I was trying to figure out when the "no's" and "impossibilities" were going to jump out, bringing our attempt to a screeching halt.

We floated out of the financial office and met with the nurse once more. I was rubella non-immune and would have to receive the vaccination again. The procedure could be done three months following my vaccination, which will be August. Just three months away! August! I love August! We practically skipped out of the office. We hugged and kissed our way down the elevator. We found an Olive Garden close by to have dinner, and we celebrated the good news. We couldn't quit smiling and laughing. We were genuinely overjoyed!

On our way home I began to filter through the paperwork and recalculated the figures to compare what the financial office had told us. I wanted to make sure we understood her correctly and didn't miss something important. We also made the decision to keep this a secret for the time being because we are still three months away, and so much could go wrong in that length of time. We knew this by experience. We couldn't handle this being public knowledge and then not be able to afford it or to have some other problem pop up and steal our chance away. This will be the hardest secret to keep! I wanted to shout our grand secret to every person I passed. God is finally moving in our behalf.

I can't help but to feel so humbled by the current events, my sweet baby. If it were not for my friend's tragedy I may have never received this opportunity. When I look back on my unbelievable journey, I stand amazed at where God has brought me from and how He brought these things about. I marvel at His goodness and faithfulness to us. My anticipation for you is now greater than ever before, and things are feeling more real than ever. My faith is being rebuilt as it replaces the doubt. My heart is filling with joy as the sadness trickles out. I give thanks to God as I bubble over with happiness and gratitude for what He has done in our lives. I may not sleep tonight, dear child, but the insomnia will be that of elation. Enjoy heaven now, precious angel, for you will be coming to us very soon.

With a heart bursting with love and anticipation,

Mommy

September 10th, 2000

To our sweet angel baby,

It has been a long four months full of anticipation. Our hopes for the future have risen to unbelievable heights. Soon after our first visit in Charleston we received a check in the mail from a credit agency. Even though it had a high interest rate, it would be a quick but temporary fix to the financial dilemma we had for our procedure. The check would cover what my insurance would not. So we thankfully cashed it and put it into our savings.

As part of the prerequisites, we had to attend an orientation at the clinic and be evaluated by a psychologist to deem us fit to proceed with IVF. We successfully took care of those incidentals during our three-month wait, taking caution not to expose our secret to our family. Only a few people knew and that was because they had to. We needed several people to care for Hope and we had to be explicit with them so they would know why and how to reach us.

August finally came and it was time to start the first phase of many to bring you to us. On August 13, 2000, I started my first round of fertility drug injections. I would have to take this daily until enough eggs would be produced and mature enough for a retrieval process. We were so excited to get to this point, but also nervous as to what to expect and what the injections would feel like.

Your daddy was too scared to give me the injections himself as he has a fear of needles (especially long ones!). A friend of mine who also happens to be a nurse attends our church. We asked Ronda if she would mind helping us out with some of the injections. She hesitantly agreed. She had limited experience with intramuscular injections, but she would do whatever she could to help us out.

The night of the 13th, we were at church and the three of us met secretly in one of the classrooms. Your daddy came to offer moral support as well as to observe in case he would have to give an injection in the event of an emergency. We all took a deep breath as I carefully mixed the drugs and drew them up into the syringe. The two-inch needle looked like it would reach my bone! I lay down on the floor as I tried to relax my tense muscles, knowing this would make the injection easier for all of us. I positioned myself on my side, facing your daddy and burying my face in his lap as I held onto his hand with an unrelenting grip. The tension in the room mounted. All three of us were petrified of what was about to take place. Especially me! That's when we all started to chuckle nervously and pray. "In Jesus' name, In Jesus' name, dear Jesus, please help us get through this." We anxiously giggled this prayer over and over, hoping divine intervention would come down upon us giving Ronda the courage to administer the injection and me the strength to receive it. I felt her hands shaking, which did absolutely nothing for my anxiety. I encouraged her to just do it and get it over with—we would all feel much better afterwards.

"Besides, it is better to give than to receive," I joked. I tried desperately to relax as I felt her aiming the needle toward my backside as if preparing to throw a dart at the bull's eye. The next thing I knew, the needle had been painlessly inserted and my muscle cramped as it received the medication.

"It didn't hurt," I exclaimed. "It didn't hurt!" I was so relieved, I nearly cried. We laughed and hugged, as all of us still shook with relief of it being over. This was just the first of many injections to come. It would take a total of nine injections for my eggs to fully mature and ripen for retrieval.

Ronda continued to help us, as well as several nurses that I worked with. Some were better than others, but in all, the injections were not too bad. My hips were very sore and the heating pad became my best friend. My abdomen got very tender and bloated as my ovaries expanded with an overabundance of eggs. Near the end of my injections it became a trial just to walk with all of these newly acquired aches and pains. I kept my eyes set on my goal and the symptoms became irrelevant.

I had a total of four ultrasounds and four lab draws to closely monitor my status during the nine days of injections. These were done at Dr. T.'s office to cut down on some of the traveling that we had to do.

On August 19th, Dr. Y. requested we come to Charleston for this ultrasound because I could possibly be ready to move forward. He found I was developing many eggs, but he wanted to give them three more days. I was in a panic because we used up the fertility drugs he initially thought we would need and we bought those at a greatly discounted price. To make matters worse, this was a Saturday. Where would I get these drugs so quickly? Who would carry them? How were we going to pay for them? Dr. Y. wrote us out a prescription and gave us the name of a local pharmacy that would carry the medication.

We made our way back to the car and called the pharmacy on our cell phone, praying they would have the medication in stock. They had it! The pharmacist gave us directions to their store and we were able to navigate ourselves to the pharmacy without complication. He handed us our three days worth of medication along with its hefty price tag of three hundred and twelve dollars! We wrote a check in good faith and gratefully took the medication, knowing the priceless gift it was going to help us obtain.

We decided now was the time to tell our parents. My parents already knew some of the details because of keeping Hope for us, so we just needed to let them know that this was it.

We asked your daddy's parents to stay after church one night, because we had something to talk to them about. We sat on the front pew of the church and sprung the news that I had been on fertility drugs and if all went well, in a few days we would undergo a procedure to become pregnant and would likely not be in church on Sunday. They were ecstatic! We shared happy hugs, then joined hands and prayed for God to have His hand on us and to bring about our miracle.

After another ultrasound and blood work on August 22nd, we finally received word to give my HCG injection precisely at 9:30 p.m. that evening. That would mean my eggs would be harvested at 7:00 a.m. on the 24th. We had to be timely with the injection because there is a small window of opportunity to successfully retrieve the eggs before my body would release them on its own.

We were thrilled to be moving on to the next step. We made it through another portion without anything going wrong. Just one wrong thing at the wrong time could cause the whole cycle to come to an abrupt, unsuccessful end.

We spent the night at the Marriott in Charleston, because we had to arrive at the hospital at 6:45 a.m. I was not a bit nervous. Instead, I was filled with excitement. We had to stop at admissions to check in and get registered. We also had to pay for the procedure up front and the insurance would reimburse what it needed to. I then was taken to a small recovery area where the nurses greeted us and made us feel right at home. They had me change into a gown and gave me warmed blankets to help me feel comfortable. They started an IV that would be necessary for pain medications and sedation. The staff was marvelous and did all in their ability to make us feel at ease.

The time came for me to be wheeled into the operating room where the procedure would take place. Thankfully, your daddy was able to come along to provide the much-needed support at this time. My nurse reassured me that she would be in charge of keeping me comfortable. She said that if I showed any signs of pain she would administer pain medication and promised to do her best at keeping me pain-free. She jokingly added that the most common side effect is snoring. She always makes the patient's husband give his word that he won't tell his wife how loud she snored! I said if that was all I had to worry about, that was fine with me.

My legs were placed in special stirrups. Quite a humiliating position to be in, with a room full of people present. The embryologist waited at a half door that was between the OR suite and his lab. Dr. Y. prepared me for what was about to take place by reviewing the steps of the procedure with us. Afterward, the nurse administered a sedative. With oxygen and monitors lulling me, I quickly drifted off into sleep. I woke once, pulling at the oxygen. Apparently one of the drugs I was given is notorious for making one's nose itch. I did flinch with pain several times, but the nurse kept her word and I was promptly made comfortable again. That is all I remember of my retrieval.

I was roused out of my sleep in the OR and told to scoot back over to my cart, upon which I was wheeled back to the recovery area and monitored for several hours. I was given the great news that Dr. Y. retrieved twenty-two eggs! That was twenty-two possibilities! He later joked with me that if I ever wanted to become an egg donor to give him a call.

Now it was time for your daddy to go to the lab to give them a specimen that was required to inject the eggs. He met me back in the recovery room, and after he saw that all was well with me, he decided to go back to the hotel to collect our belongings and get us checked out. Right after he left, the nurse received a phone call from the lab. With a bewildered look on her face, the nurse asked, "Mrs. Donham, where is your husband? The lab needs another specimen—the first was not enough."

Panic set in as an avalanche of fear buried me. We came this far and now back to the same problem again? I gave them our cell phone number and the number at the hotel to try to catch him. I worried and prayed until he returned. When he arrived back at the lab, he had the same sinking feeling, too. Were we going to go through all of this for nothing? It jolted us back into reality.

After my recovery time was up, I made my way to the restroom with my throbbing abdomen, where I changed my clothes to head home. I was very sore! We went home with a cautious attitude. We anxiously waited for a phone call the next morning from our embryologist to see how many babies we had—if any.

The next morning, we were awakened by the phone ringing. It was the embryologist. He stated that he attempted to fertilize twelve eggs after our procedure, but only four of them "took." He said he was having a difficult time with them, but he would attempt to fertilize more that day if the eggs were mature enough.

My heart quivered as I realized that this might come to a terrible end. I had to be prepared within if this was not meant to be. Your daddy was crushed. He carried a heavy burden that day, feeling that if things were not successful it would primarily be because of the problem he had. We tried to stay focused on the fact that at least we did have four. It only takes one to achieve a pregnancy, and it could be one of our four that we already had.

I also discussed my painfully tight abdomen with the embryologist. I was sent to our local hospital right away for emergency lab work to be obtained. It seemed that I was going into hyperstimulation syndrome from the retrieval. My body was trying to compensate for all of the fluid that was aspirated from my ovaries, causing an imbalance in my lab work and ascites (fluid in the abdomen). This could also bring things to a devastating halt. Fortunately, my lab work was "on the fence" between what it should or should not be. They continued to watch me closely until the fluid went down and my labs returned to normal.

The next morning we received another phone call from the embryologist stating he was able to fertilize six more eggs and one other "took" from the day before over night. Our first four also continued to grow. That made a total of eleven babies! When I got off the phone, I flew down the stairs holding a pillow tightly against my tender belly, and delivered the exciting news to your daddy while he still lay in bed. He broke down in tears, crying with relief. He was so happy! It lifted the heavy burden he had carried the day prior. We immediately prayed for God to keep His hands on our babies and to help them grow healthy and strong.

We were now scheduled for the embryo transfer on August 27, 2000, which was a Sunday. We stayed at Embassy Suites the night before, courtesy of your Aunt Kathy, and had a restful evening. I also had to start my progesterone injections that evening to help my uterus support my impending pregnancy. We woke early and ate a huge breakfast before leaving for the hospital. We arrived at the clinic at 8 a.m. for the transfer. We were to go to the same area as before when we had the retrieval done. After breakfast I drank liquids, because I was to have a full bladder for the procedure. Apparently, I did a superb job at drinking because I was so full I could barely stand it! I talked the nurse into letting me partially empty my bladder prior to the procedure because it was getting very uncomfortable.

I was dressed in my gown and again draped with warm blankets as I lay on my cart waiting to go to the operating room for the procedure. Dr. B., who was another specialist in the clinic, would be performing the transfer that day. Dr. O. arrived before Dr. B. and he showed us a picture of the four embryos he had chosen for the transfer. We oohed and aahed over the picture as we gazed at them in amazement. One of these babies could be you! Would we get more than one baby? We chattered on about whether these embryos were boys or girls and we told them how we felt we were going to have a baby boy because of all the dreams we had. There was even some discussion of your name and how your Grammy wanted you named after my dad. It all started to spin around in my head just thinking of the possibilities I now faced. Dr. O. then informed us that we were his worst case in all of the years he had practiced. He said that it took him nearly three hours to inject our eggs, when it should have only taken forty minutes. He said the sperm quality was very poor and he had to "go fishing" to search for the best specimens to produce favorable embryos. I then felt even more blessed, realizing what a miracle all of this had been for us to make it so far.

When Dr. B. arrived, Dr. O. showed him the picture and they discussed my fate. They walked over to my bedside and with a doctor on either side of me, they debated my future as if I were not even there! I threw my head from side to side trying to keep up with this head-spinning yet detrimental conversation about me and my baby(ies). Dr. O. felt that all four should be implanted for a successful chance at one baby while Dr. B. was concerned with my young age and felt that all four could take and I would have quads! So depending on who you listened to, it sounded like an all or nothing chance. Who was right? Dr. B. held his chin in a concerned fashion while talking to himself, but every now and then lifting his eyes to ask Dr. O. or me another question.

He muttered to himself, "Triplets, twins, hmmm, she is tall enough to carry more than one." Then he turned my way and asked, "Are you sure you couldn't reduce a multiple pregnancy?" I told him there was no way I could have an abortion. How could anyone create life to just destroy it again? Then He turned to Dr. O. again and asked, "All four?" That's when I became panic stricken and my heart felt as if it would leap out of my chest. With all of the uncertainty in the room, I was not sure if I was going to end up with a herd of babies or any baby at all.

I was captivated by fear. I felt like an unsuspecting lab rat being set up for some freak experiment. Finally I gasped, "Look, you guys are the professionals here. I trust whatever decision you make on my behalf. Do what your instincts are telling you to do."

Dr. O., who was in favor of all four turned and said, "How old are you again?"

I emphatically replied, "Twenty-seven years old."

He said, "Oh, I didn't realize you were that young—we better go with three." A compromise was made. I believe God intervened again by giving the doctors wisdom in managing our case. We all sighed a breath of relief.

I then was wheeled into the OR suite where I was placed back in the embarrassing pose in those stirrups. My nurse kindly covered me in a discreet fashion until the procedure began. With my mind off of the alarming conversation I had just witnessed, it was now turned back to my painfully full bladder. I was assured that the procedure would take just a few moments and I could relieve myself shortly after that. The doctor inserted the speculum and it scraped my cervix. I have a very sensitive cervix, so the insertion caused bleeding. Dr. B. dabbed and swabbed my cervix, attempting to get the bleeding to stop. It took forty long minutes before things were suitable for transfer. I broke out into a cold sweat from my bladder being excruciatingly full. Your daddy and my nurse held my hands and wiped my brow as they encouraged me and told me to hang in there, hoping things would be over soon.

The pressure from the ultrasound wand over my bladder was immense. I was breathing hard and I warned Dr. B. that when he removed the speculum I was not responsible for what would happen. I told him to watch his shoes because a great flood could be coming his way! He laughed and reminded me that worse things have happened. Dr. O. handed over the syringe with my babies to Dr. B., and they were successfully implanted to the safety and security of my welcoming womb. I instantly felt pregnant!

The speculum was removed without incident (thankfully) and I was carefully transferred back to the recovery area, where I had to lay in a backward tilt with my hips elevated on pillows. This would give the embryos a chance to attach themselves to my uterine lining. Still in great discomfort, my nurse offered a bedpan while I lay practically upside down in my awkward position. Her heart was in the right place, but imagine being on a bedpan while trying to pee uphill. It wasn't going to happen for me, no matter how painful my bladder was. Not to mention that my bladder normally suffers from stage fright and a room full of people didn't help matters any. Finally, the bed was flattened, all staff left the room, and while hidden behind curtain number two, I was able to prop myself temporarily on my elbows and give myself the relief I had waited all morning for.

Now came our two-hour wait with hips still propped in the air before we could go home. Our nurse was super sweet and we found her to be a fellow Christian. She plopped down on the bed beside mine and held conversation with us about our story, church and the Lord. It was so wonderful to have this woman of faith providing us with care and encouragement. It made the time fly by. Not to mention how it lifted our spirits.

It was now time to make our way on our long journey home. My nurse gave us both a big heart-felt hug as she helped me out of the wheelchair and into the car, promising to keep us in her prayers. I went home and put myself on three days of bed rest, giving our babies the best of chances to implant. I rubbed my tummy, thanking God for all three of my babies everyday.

That placed us in the period of time called "the two-week wait." This is the longest two weeks a hopefully expectant couple ever faces. The three days of bed rest were long enough on their own. Now we had eleven more days to go! That was an absolute eternity! Hope's third birthday was upon us, which was fun and provided us with some respite. We had her party at a local zoo and we celebrated the day away while I kept my bloated tummy a secret. Then it was back to waiting again.

Desperately trying to find salvation for our stricken minds, we decided to make a spur of the moment trip to Ocean City, Maryland. We called our doctor in Charleston and begged for approval, appealing any doubtful response with the fact that we would get more relaxation away from home. When I was given the OK, we packed our bags and jumped in the car headed for the beach. This was a much-needed mini-vacation after all of the recent drama we had been through.

I woke up early on the morning that we were leaving and tip-toed up the stairs, quietly making my way to the bathroom were I always kept a supply of pregnancy tests. Even though it was still very early, curiosity was getting the best of me and I couldn't stand it any longer. I took the pregnancy test and distracted myself as I prepared for the day's journey. All the while I kept my eyes on the clock. It was time to check the results. What if it is negative? Should I have allowed myself to do this so early? Should I just throw the test away and not look? I have to look! What if it is positive? What should I do?

Trembling, I picked up the test stick before I could talk myself out of it. My heart pounded and I held my breath as I reached for the test. Holding the stick carefully in the light, I found a faint pink line. What? A faint pink line? I turned and twisted the stick under the light to rule out a shadow, but no matter how I moved the little stick under the light, the pink line was still there. This was a sight I had never seen before. I was pregnant!

I bounced my way down the stairs and shook your daddy awake, exclaiming, "Come upstairs and look at this, I think I am pregnant!" He followed me back to the bathroom where we examined the test together, and he confirmed it in my disbelief. It just didn't seem real. I paused to see if I would wake from this glorious dream, but so far, I was still there.

We immediately made a mad dash for the telephone to call our parents and tell them our amazing news before leaving for Ocean City. We embraced, knowing this was going to be a wonderful week. Relaxation wouldn't be so hard to come by now.

We arrived at our destination where we soaked up the sun, made sand castles on the beach, and romped with Hope. We had a marvelous time together. I couldn't help but to think that this would probably be the last vacation with just the three of us. That made it even more special. Before leaving for home, we decided to take another pregnancy test just to be sure of our first result. And like the first, we watched a pink line appear. We were ecstatic!

We arrived home at the end of our two-week wait period. It was now time for us to confirm our home pregnancy tests with the already scheduled blood test. Hope and I woke up early and went to the lab at our local hospital where they drew my blood. I got a band-aid. Hope got a sticker. We anxiously drove home to wait for the result and to get my new HCG level. After several phone calls on our part, we were finally successful at finding out our results. 221! We were definitely, undeniably, absolutely, miraculously pregnant! I was so thrilled I couldn't contain myself! Without thinking I dialed one number right after another shouting, "I'm pregnant, I'm pregnant!"

After giving a brief update to the person on the phone, I would hang up as quickly as I called and repeat the scenario over and over until all of those who were waiting with us knew. Suddenly, I realized I had not told your daddy. I was so caught up in the magic of it all I had forgotten to go downstairs to wake him up! I ran down the stairs to find him awake in bed saying, "I know, I know, you're pregnant!" mocking my exuberant tone I was using on the phone. He happily told me my screaming woke him up. I bounced on the bed in excitement as we celebrated our miracle.

Our minds quickly switched gears. Now that we were truly pregnant, how many babies did we have? We could have triplets! Or twins! Or—Or—a baby! Our doctor finally called us and gave us the following statistics. We had a 55% chance of having one healthy baby, 27% chance of having healthy twins, 3% chance of having healthy triplets, and finally, a 20% chance of a miscarriage. Our thoughts then turned to prayers that God would keep our babies safe and healthy and that He would do His will.

Now I find myself having to go back to work this week. I don't know if I will be able to anchor myself down from the clouds long enough to get anything accomplished. Everyone at work is thrilled for us also. They have been very supportive of me during this long tedious process. I am ever so grateful to them for that.

We are scheduled for an ultrasound on September 20th. I am counting the days until then. I can't even imagine what it will be like to get a precious glimpse of you after all of these years of waiting. It seems so unbelievable. So far, only our parents and a few close friends know of your impending arrival. This is the most difficult secret I have ever had to keep. However, we have made the decision not to tell everyone until after the ultrasound so that we can confirm a heartbeat and also know how many babies I am carrying. We are just so thankful and appreciative that you are coming to us. We can't wait to shout it from the mountaintops. Our angel baby is on the way.

I love you with all of my heart,

Mommy

September 20, 2000

Dear angel baby,

We had our first ultrasound today and received quite a scare. We arrived at Dr. T.'s office around 7:30 a.m. to have our ultrasound done. This was to confirm our pregnancy and your heartbeat. We anxiously waited in the exam room as the nurse prepared the equipment for our scan. Dr. T. entered the room and greeted us as he sat down at the monitor and began to perform the testing. I hunched myself up on my elbows desperately trying to see the screen because I didn't want to miss that first glimpse of my baby. *And what if it is babies*? I thought.

"Dorothy! Dorothy! Breathe, honey, take a deep breath and breathe!" the nurse ordered. In all of my eagerness I didn't realize how "blown away" I really was by all of this. In my hunched position, I was panting like a runner at the end of a marathon on the verge of hyperventilation. I laughed as I realized the condition of myself and explained my well-understood excitement.

As we watched various images flicker on the screen my patience grew thinner. "Do you see my baby, Dr. T.?" He mumbled something and then informed me that he could see a yolk sac. "What do you mean?" He told me that he could not visualize an embryo, just a yolk sac. With me still not fully understanding what he was implicating, I asked for a picture from my ultrasound. He replied, "I guess, but there is really nothing there." He then said that he would send the results to Charleston and they would probably want to re-scan me at a later date. The scan came to an end with no reassurance one way or another.

We left the office quite puzzled. Your daddy left for home and I went to work. Slowly, as the excitement wore off, the information started to sink in. I wanted to be pregnant so badly and I was so overjoyed by the positive pregnancy tests I had received, I was not allowing myself to get the full impact of what the doctor had been saying. He said that he could not see my baby! But there was a yolk sac—what did that mean? Was I pregnant or not? When I got to the office I put in a call for your daddy to call me back. I then started to look information up on the Internet, only to find that you can have positive pregnancy tests and have an empty gestational sac. Was this what was happening to me?

I got up from my desk and ran to the bathroom where I absolutely fell apart. I sobbed and bawled until I got the courage to return to my desk to call Dr. Y. I made a frantic call to Charleston with a tearful plea for help.

The nurse promptly returned my call and gave me plenty of reassurance that everything was okay. She said that this is exactly what they would expect to see at this stage in the game and that they were happy and not concerned. A tremendous amount of relief poured over me as I thanked her with all of my heart for calling me back with good news.

I called your daddy back and gave him the good news to put his mind at ease, too. Now that we were comforted with the fact that I was still pregnant, our thoughts quickly went to the babies we had lost. My womb once held three precious lives and now only one clung there. After the day's events, I was so grateful to have you, but a part of me was saddened and grieved by the loss of your siblings. But God has a plan and we are in His will. We now await another ultrasound in Charleston on October 3rd. This time we will confirm your heart beat.

Please hang in there, little one, and grow strong as each precious part of you continues to develop. We anxiously await our next scan so that we can peek into your quiet little world and catch a glimpse of you. We love you so much already. Thank you for being here and for coming to us!

With much relief,
Mommy

October 6, 2000

To my dear angel baby,

Well, my sweet child, we survived another two-week wait and our fears have now subsided by the good news we received today. I am definitely pregnant with one big beautiful baby!

We made our way back to Women and Children's Hospital in Charleston. I was nervous and restless, wanting to confirm the status of my pregnancy even though I was reassured earlier that all was fine. I just had an urgent need to see it for myself and to know that you were unquestionably OK. We arrived in the office and were seated in the full waiting room. We waited—and waited—and waited. Not many other people came or went while we waited. All of us sat anxiously together as we each grew more uptight regarding our personal situations. After an hour or so passed, we learned that Dr. Y. was still in the OR with a patient and would be arriving as soon as he could make it.

Finally, we were escorted to an exam room where we continued to wait. The nurse came in and held some light conversation with us. That helped divert our attention for a short span of time. When she wasn't in the room we paced the floors and watched the clock. After three grueling hours, Dr. Y. arrived and we were hurried off to the ultrasound room.

After changing my clothes and getting positioned on the exam table, Dr. Y. entered the room, greeted us, and finally began to perform my ultrasound. We had brought a videotape to share our first peek at you with our family. The nurse placed our videotape in the machine, but said she would wait until we confirmed good news before she would record. All eyes in the room apprehensively watched the screen of black and white. The silence was broken by Dr. Y. exclaiming, "There it is! There is your baby!" We all cheered as the worry lifted from us. Dr. Y. pointed out your head and tiny little body with arms and legs budding from the appropriate positions. But most importantly, he directed our attention to the center of your fragile little body. It was then that we saw your beautiful heart beating strongly and pounding away in your chest! Then it happened, a moment in time I will never forget. Dr. Y. reached over and turned the volume up on the machine and we heard your heartbeat for the very first time. Tears filled our eyes with happiness and amazement as we listened to the cadence of your heart rhythm beating endlessly within my tummy. You were here! Instantly I fell in love! I was swept away with adoration for you.

We admired you a little longer and even caught you moving once. Dr. Y. also turned on a color monitor and showed us the blood flow passing through your umbilical cord, placenta, heart, and body. It was so amazing. Even though we knew when you were conceived, you measured ahead of schedule! We all gushed about how big you are. You could all but feel the buttons popping off our shirts as we swelled with pride. And it was as if our doctor and nurse were viewing a baby for the very first time, too. We were all so awestruck and ecstatic with your arrival. When the scan came to an end, the nurse handed me my videotape and it felt as if she handed me a valuable treasure. We couldn't wait to show our family!

After I got dressed, Dr. Y. came back into the room and gave us both huge bear hugs. We hugged back with deep gratitude in our hearts. We told him that we were forever indebted to him. I joked that if I were rich, I would buy him anything in the world. He replied that just a picture would do. I smiled and told him we could definitely manage that. They both assured us that they would not abandon us now. We were to keep in touch with any questions we may have along the way and to of course keep them updated on our condition. We were also told that we could finally stop the painful progesterone injections that had helped support this pregnancy.

Including the fertility drugs I had taken in the beginning, I have had a total of fifty-two intramuscular injections to become pregnant and then to support it. I have the sore, knot-ridden hips to prove it, too!

It felt as if a heavy weight was released from us and I felt lighter than air. A new sense of joy and accomplishment filled my being. I floated back to the car as we thanked God once again for being so faithful and good to us.

We have waited so long for this moment in time. Our journey to this point has been a very long one. All of the pain we have suffered as we ached for you has tremendously diminished. What healing you have brought to our lives, sweet angel. For the first time, I feel complete. Our family will be rounded out and complete, too. I remain in a dreamlike state as I try to comprehend that you are tucked safely in my womb.

I feel like I have started a brand new life. I now see things from a fresh perspective. Just thinking that I have a part of me and a part of your daddy growing inside of me brings such an exciting feeling. At one time we thought we would never be able to experience such a privilege. You are such a miracle!

Thank you for coming to us, sweet baby. We have prayed for you for so long. As we pass each milestone, we long to hold you more and more. You are our priceless treasure, sweetheart!

I love you, my miracle,

Mommy

October 25, 2000

Dear sweet angel baby,

We had our first official visit with our doctor. It is so strange for us now that we are pregnant, because we are now treated as normal, everyday patients. However, our not-so-normal conception has everyone intrigued.

Our first appointment was actually with a nurse practitioner. She took a thorough health history from both of us and went over a vast amount of teaching and instructions for new parents. It was slightly overwhelming, but very helpful. She spoke to us about what tests would be scheduled during my pregnancy and why they would be of benefit.

We chose to decline an amniocentesis because we didn't want to jeopardize this delicate pregnancy in any way. Nearly one out of two hundred miscarry and we would not take that chance. In addition, even if a health issue arose, we planned on keeping you and loving you the same. We also declined the A.F.P. screening. We felt it would provide us with more unneeded worry. It has a high false-positive rate and we already knew we didn't want an amniocentesis. Another observation that was made was because of your unusually incredible conception we would have a level three ultrasound to inspect every part of you thoroughly for any problems. Also, because of your cousin Ashley's major heart defect, they felt it necessary for you to have a fetal echo when the time is right.

With all of the planning behind us, it was time for our physical examination. After the nurse was completed she brought a doppler into the room to attempt to find your heartbeat through my abdomen.

She applied cold jelly to my abdomen and brushed the doppler from side to side over my belly, scrambling to find a heartbeat. Suddenly, a loud *swish, swish, swish, swish* filled the room as your heart played its tune through the speaker. A sigh of relief escaped me as we reached another milestone. It sounded so fast and so strong. It was very comforting to know things were still OK.

We are so elated about this new pregnancy. We thank God several times each day for this miracle pregnancy and our miracle baby that I am carrying. I have never felt happier (or more tired) than I am right now. I feel so connected to you already. Even though you are barely here. We know how thin the line was when it came to our attempt to have you. We are so thankful, dear baby. We still think of your siblings, too. A part of us grieves for them daily. Even though we know it was God's will, they were still our children. Not only did we lose the two that briefly shared my womb with you, the previous eight had ceased to grow in the lab and we were unable to keep them for a future pregnancy.

One particular day while mourning the two I miscarried, I decided to give them both a name. Even though they never made it into this world, I felt they deserved an identity and something we could relate to. We chose unisex names, not knowing if they were a boy or a girl. One we named Madison, meaning "gift of God." The other we named Gabriel, meaning "angel; devoted to God." I also wrote a poem in their memory:

> One day in heaven,
> the Lord chose three of His most precious angels
> to perform a very important task.
> I have a special job
> for each one of you
> that will require your love
> and unselfishness to do.
> For you'll have to turn in
> your halo and your wings
> because very soon

you'll be tiny human beings.
On Earth a longing couple prayed
parents they should be.
Now in My own timing,
I see fit to send them three.
You'll bring their hearts great joy
and fill their lives with love abound.
All because their heartbreak
will be turned around.
So show your love and compassion
and go where I send.
Then again in My perfect timing
your job will come to an end.
At My chosen time
your wings again you'll put on.
Tears they will shed
when they learn that you have gone.
But don't worry, precious angels,
My work is not finished yet.
For one of you I shall leave behind
to be their heaven sent.

In loving memory of our two angels who found their wings.
September 2000

This poem will be displayed in your room along with angel wings
bearing the names of your siblings and a picture of that very first ultra
sound from Dr. T.'s office.

I find my every waking thought turned to you. Isn't it funny how
when we suffered from infertility and even now in pregnancy you
hold me spellbound? You are one special baby. I also find myself
doing everything very carefully. From my diet to my activities, I am
very cautious about every move I make in your behalf. I would never
want to do anything that would risk this precious pregnancy. You are
priceless to us! I want to give you every chance that I can.

I am feeling many changes in my body now because of you. My belly had already been very bloated after having I.V.F. and the fertility drugs associated with it. So really, I started out with a bit of a "potbelly." Very early on I noticed blue veins creeping over my breasts and tummy as the blood volume in my body increased. It was comforting seeing my body finally doing what it should to support a pregnancy. I feel very tired all of the time and I always want to eat, eat and eat! I don't really have nausea unless I have an empty stomach. I am amazed with each and every little change my body makes to accommodate it's new boarder who is working hard inside of me. It is a very exciting time.

My body is not the only thing making changes, little one. We are finally starting to think about changes we need to make for you. We are in the midst of plans to build a new home to provide for our growing family. We are also placing our thoughts on your future needs.

During my infertility, I would longingly gaze at baby items when we went shopping. There was one thing in particular that I admired and had set my heart on for you. It was a round white canopy crib with a flowing white canopy that showered down and gracefully landed on the floor. I was smitten by it. Every time I saw it, my heart would ache for you. I would rub my hand over the plush comforter and imagine what it would look like in my home with my angel baby enveloped in the softness of the blankets tucked neatly in the center of this "hope chest." There were times that I would see it and literally burst into tears from the devastation I had faced. I remember one particular instant when I was shopping in that store for a baby gift and the clerk approached me and asked, "Are you pregnant?" As if I shouldn't be in that department if I were not.

I glared back at her and said just as rudely, "If you have to know, we can't have children—not that it's any of your business!" I spun around on my heels and stomped away. The last thing I remember was seeing her gasp as she tossed her head around hoping no one had witnessed the embarrassing predicament she put herself in.

One day recently, your daddy and I went shopping again. I told him since I was now officially pregnant, I wanted to look at "my" crib again. We happily pranced to the baby department and found no crib. It would have been hard to miss, but I scoured the area aisle by aisle just to make sure and still—no crib! I was now alarmed. I frantically found a clerk and asked her where the beautiful round canopy crib was and she politely informed me that they were discontinued. "What?" I gasped as I tried not to break down in tears. After a moment of shock, she quickly remembered that there had been one put away in the stock room and she kindly offered to go and check for us. I warned your daddy that if it was there, we would have to purchase it. There was no way I would take a chance of losing it again.

The clerk reappeared with a smile stating they had the last one in the stock room. Before your daddy could say anything I quickly stammered, "We'll take it!" So there we were—six weeks pregnant and buying a crib. We were truly stepping out in faith because that was even before we confirmed your heartbeat. I yearned for a baby for over four years to put in that crib and now that the baby was coming—I was going to have it. I am sure it will be gorgeous in your new room. I can't wait to see it in the nursery!

Well, my love, it has been an eventful day. I love you with all of my heart and I am savoring each and every precious moment with you. I will have a lifetime of wonderful memories of this time together. You're my angel baby!

With a heart full of love,
Mommy

November 29, 2000

To our lovely little treasure,
This morning I woke up to a big surprise—my tummy! I couldn't believe my eyes! Yesterday I carried my little "potbelly." Today I carry a big belly! Somehow I have literally doubled in size overnight. I don't know how it happened, but it did. Now when I lie down, I can easily feel my uterus in my abdomen without pushing and prodding. Everyone at church commented on how I have grown without me saying anything. It is very noticeable now. I am so proud of my growing tummy; I can show you off now. I am still between my clothes and maternity clothes though. Just keep growing and growing, dear baby!

Oh, sweet angel, we have reached so many important goals in our pregnancy successfully. We breezed right through the first trimester. The fatigue and the little bit of queasiness that I once had has now faded away and I am feeling happy and energetic. I give thanks to God for withholding the morning sickness and other common side effects of early pregnancy.

At about ten and a half weeks, we rented a professional doppler off of the Internet so that we could periodically check in on you and enjoy you in your hidden sanctuary. It arrived a few days later on our front porch and I was the first to find the package. I snatched it up and hid in the bathroom with it. I quickly tore into the box spilling out the contents. After adjusting a few things I anxiously lay on the bathroom floor sweeping the doppler's wand over my lower abdomen in search of any sound from my baby. *Swish, swish, swish, swish*! There it was—your heart beating away right were we left off before. I gleefully called for your daddy to reveal the surprise to him. When he entered the room, your heartbeat greeted him. We sat there in awe as we listened intently to every bump and thud you made.

My next adventure with the doppler was the telephone. I would lie on the couch and search for your heartbeat (you are a squirmy little thing!). As soon as it was located, I quickly dialed the phone to let a family member or friend hear. It was so wonderful being able to share such a special moment with them. Especially the first time I did it. Everyone got to experience this miracle with me. That has meant a great deal to me. I am so happy I have been able to share you with our family. By the way, I check in on you every day.

Another major event occurred on November 18th. I slept through the whole night without having to pee! I know that doesn't sound like a big deal, but when you've had interrupted sleep for weeks on end, it becomes a special occasion. I guess it is God's way of preparing new mothers for the sleepless nights ahead. That's OK. I will gladly lose sleep for you any day. Even though sleeping through the night meant a lot to me, that wasn't the major event I was referring to. The major event was that we felt you move for the first time!

After waking up early that morning, I discovered my uncomfortably full bladder that was bloating my belly. Just then, I felt a squirmy little flip-flop just beneath my navel. It certainly grabbed my attention. And just as I began to think about what I just felt—It happened again! Now I was curious. I suspiciously poked and jabbed my abdomen stirring my unsuspecting boarder. I received two more fluttery movements. I was so excited, without thinking I yelled, "Jody—wake up!" He sprung straight out of bed with a panic-ridden expression over his face. After he awoke and realized what I wanted, he got to experience the miracle of a lifetime. He felt you move twice. That was one of the most spectacular moments of our life. It seemed to verify the fact that we have a tiny precious life growing inside of me. I have been overjoyed!

I was only fourteen and a half weeks pregnant that day. I know that my thin stature and full bladder is what allowed us to experience that joy so early on. Since then I have felt you move several times.

You deliver gentle pokes and prods that come several days in between. I do notice them a little easier now than from the first time I felt you. Something so amazing happens when I feel you move. I instantly give a large uncontainable smile. My emotion of happiness seems to be connected right to you.

I have enjoyed every second of this pregnancy thus far. It truly has been a remarkable journey. Now we anxiously await our next ultrasound. We can't wait to be able to see how you have grown and to confirm your gender (we still think you're a boy). We love you so much sweet baby. You're our precious gift.

I love you, my darling baby,

Mommy

December 21, 2000

To my sweet baby boy,

Yes, my angel baby, you're a boy! Today we had our much-anticipated ultrasound. We anxiously watched the clock for our appointment time to roll around as I continued to drink liquids to fill my bladder for the test. We were slightly nervous because we wanted to make sure that you were healthy. We were scheduled to have a level three ultrasound because of the way you were conceived. My doctor didn't want to leave anything to chance and we wanted to be fully aware if there were any problems to be found.

After what seemed to be an eternal wait in the waiting room, we were finally called in to the exam room by a technician. We had brought another videotape and even our camcorder in case that wouldn't work, hoping to capture this special moment once again for a keepsake. To our dismay, the machine they used that day was not capable of recording, nor would they allow us to videotape for legal reasons. I was disappointed, but my focus quickly turned back to you and what we were about to see.

The technician squeezed the cold jelly on my lower abdomen and scanned over my pregnant uterus. Immediately, we were able to see images of you race across the screen. I was breathless! I couldn't believe I had just seen your arm. It was fully developed! Then a long leg! And your head—wait—there was your face! Look at that face! You look like your daddy! Oh! There are your fingers moving to your mouth—then you began to suck on them. We watched in amazement as this wonder continued to present itself before us.

The technician scanned every inch of you. We witnessed your

bones, organs, brain, and heart. We watched you take in fluid and swallow it. We were able to follow its path to your stomach. What a miracle you are! You measure about eight inches and weigh approximately thirteen ounces. And I can't begin to explain how much I love every one of those inches and ounces!

Then she asked us the question. "Would you like to know the sex of your baby?" Of course we did! We believed we already knew, we just needed a confirmation of our belief.

From the day we learned we were pregnant, we counted the seconds until we could confirm your gender. You see, for the past four years we have had dreams of a large beautiful baby boy that has haunted us and intensified our longing for you. Anytime anyone made a reference to my pregnancy or my future pregnancy, it was always regarding a boy. Your Grammy was on a long distance phone call to an insurance representative whom she found to be a fellow Christian. She asked her to pray that we would conceive. She told my mom that she would gladly pray and felt the Lord had already spoke to her heart saying that we would give birth to a child and it would be a boy. Then for fun we checked a Chinese conception calendar. And you guessed it! A boy! We have always felt in our hearts that you would be a boy. So when the sonographer asked us if we wanted to know, we both excitedly shouted, "Yes!"

As she carefully scanned over your tiny body, she announced, "It looks like you have a boy!" I thought I would burst with pride! We cheered and hugged with our "we knew its." My face radiated with the widest smile it ever produced. I knew I was glowing as I basked in the sheer bliss of it all. My dreams had been prophetic and now were being fulfilled. I was awestruck once again. I'm getting my baby boy! My angel baby is here.

It took three people and about an hour and a half to complete the scan. The printer was broken so we only got a picture of your foot and one of your face. It looks a little alien-like, but we think you are gorgeous. Afterward, we left the office knowing we had a healthy baby boy tucked safely in my womb. As soon as we got home, we called everyone to tell them our wonderful news that you are healthy and yes—a baby boy!

My dreams have come true. I have a healthy baby boy on the way. I am already so in love with you. I can't wait to meet you and wrap my arms around you. I don't know if I will ever let you go. I guess it's time to pick out a name for you now that we know you're a boy.

I love you, joy of my life,

Mommy

December 27, 2000

To my precious baby boy,

Hello, my angel baby. We have had a wonderful holiday knowing you are on the way. My tummy is growing and you are more active than ever. Over the past two weeks I have noticed that you are moving more. These movements are much stronger than before, although they are still gentle. You are growing so rapidly, sweetheart.

It still never fails to make me smile. As soon as I feel a little bump or flutter my face uncontrollably lights up. Even in the middle of the night. I have an overwhelming urge to share this phenomenon with others as well. When I am around strangers I have to fight the urge to not grab their hand and place it on my belly as you kick and squirm.

I want to say, "Can you believe that is my baby doing that?" When I am in bed at night, I will even pick up your daddy's hand while he is sleeping and place it over you as you flip and turn trying to get comfortable. It is something so special that's just meant to be shared.

I found something very special with you that I absolutely treasure. I lie down and rub my hands briskly in a circular motion over my belly while I say, "Mommy loves you, baby boy." Almost instantly you squirm and jab at me in response, letting me know you hear me and feel my touch. That is such a priceless moment. It deepens our bond and love to immeasurable levels.

I am also getting fat and loving it! I am finally unmistakably pregnant in my clothes. Most of my weight gain has been in my belly and it appears that I am carrying you low. However, a few people have politely told me that my backside is getting wide. That is one piece of information I could have honestly lived without. I did notice in my first trimester that my hips, thighs and backside were getting noticeably "thicker" and that I could pinch up fat in places that I couldn't before. At first I was alarmed knowing that this wouldn't magically melt away when you are born. Now I rest in the reassurance that my body is doing what it should to care for you.

My weight gain had only been a pound or two between appointments, but today I gained a whopping seven pounds! But since my last appointment my belly "popped out." And of course I ate myself through Thanksgiving and Christmas. I must admit that temptation got the best of me and I cheated a lot as my weight clearly tattled on me. Another noteworthy milestone is that I started leaking colostrum. My body is preparing to feed you. I can't believe all of the intricate details I have been able to witness as my body changes for you.

We checked out well at our appointment today, but I have been having some contractions periodically since sixteen weeks of pregnancy. I attributed these to my enlarging and now weighty uterus. I mentioned these to the nurse and as I lay down upon the table I happened to have one. My uterus bunched up into a hard knot peaking in the center like a mountain. These were painless contractions, but they did feel unusual as this muscle would tighten and knot up within me. The nurse palpated them and it lasted for nearly fifty seconds. That was more than they would like so my doctor decided to investigate a little further.

I was given an internal exam and everything checked out fine. This was also reason enough to perform another ultrasound to make sure all was well within your hidden world. Although a little worried about the circumstances, we were glad to have an opportunity to peek in on you again. When they placed the wand upon my tummy, we caught you sucking your thumb! It was absolutely precious. We then saw you pucker your mouth up like a fish and swallow fluid as it spilled to your stomach. We watched your heartbeat and your bladder fill. You are so amazing. I can't believe how you have changed in just a week's time. You are so much bigger now! You are going to be beautiful. From what we can tell, I think you look like your daddy. You date one week and two days ahead of schedule. Once again, the machine was broken so we did not afford any pictures for our scant collection. The exam proved favorable and to our relief all looked well.

I was also tested for a urinary tract infection to make sure that was not the culprit of these untimely contractions. My result for that was negative, too. So I was sent home and told to monitor these cautiously if they became frequent or of great intensity or duration. I was also to call if any bleeding is noted. Thankfully, I feel well and do not feel threatened. My doctor also feels my body is trying to adjust to the heavier weight and changes that are occurring. We are very excited to meet you, but take your time to grow healthy and strong.

By the way, we think we have a name for you. We chose "Jayden" because it means "Jehovah has heard." I couldn't give you a more valuable gift than a name that proclaims the testimony of the miracle that you are and gives all of the glory to God. Your middle name will be "Bryan," after your grandfather, "Poppy." That is his middle name also. He was named after your great-great-grandfather. So you will be given the privilege to carry on a legacy within our family.

I love you, angel,

Mommy

January 15, 2001

To my precious angel baby boy,

Oh, Jayden, we have had quite a terrifying scare. On Sunday, January 7th, we went to church and went about our day as we normally would. Afterward, we went to lunch with our friends Christy and Richard. All seemed fine even though I noticed a few contractions sporadically throughout the day. When we got home, I undressed from my church clothes and did a few things around the house. These bothersome contractions still made themselves known to me. Your daddy was taking a nap, so I quietly went upstairs to the couch to assess the situation a little closer.

As I lay there with my hands spread intently over my abdomen, I felt the contractions coming, making my belly rock hard. You didn't seem to like the squeeze you were getting as the contraction caused my uterus to entangle around you. You struggled and kicked through the contraction until its grip gradually freed from you, giving you your sought after space again. As I monitored myself I grew increasingly worried. The second hand passed by with no change in my condition. The contractions lasted thirty to seventy-five seconds and came every five minutes. "This can't be right," I thought. So I watched a little longer and nothing changed. One contraction would come with just as much intensity and duration as the one that had only gone minutes before.

Now I was truly concerned. Nervously, I shouted for your daddy to come to my side. Sensing the scared tone in my voice, he jumped out of bed and ran up the stairs. When he arrived, we observed the contractions together. Something was not right. My instincts told me

97

to grab the doppler, so I could check your heart rate and make sure you were doing all right. I counted your heartbeats as I listened through the speaker. That's when it happened. A contraction came and your heart rate slowed. Your heart was previously beating at a strong 150's range and now plummeted down to 103 and 104 beats per minute. The contractions and your heart rate seemed to battle amongst each other as you struggled against the pressure inside of my uterus. Terror shot through me! Tears instantly flowed down my quivering cheeks. My heart pounded and my hands trembled. I feared the worst.

In a nightmare-like state, I grabbed for the phone and dialed the doctor on call. I desperately tried to settle my breathing and attempted to choke back the tears to explain to the doctor the details that were unfolding. He asked if I was bleeding which, thankfully, I was not. He then kindly explained that experience was telling him that this would probably stop on its own and to just watch the contractions. At that moment I hoped his experience would start speaking to me because I was feeling far from calm, especially with your heart rate dropping. That was explained away as a "normal reaction" from you to your changing environment. As long as your heart rate didn't drop below one hundred, it was okay. I thought one hundred and three was awfully close. This was my precious baby we were talking about!

Then the bomb dropped on me. The doctor's voice boomed in my ears as an explosion of bad news rained down over my ears. I was informed that being only twenty-two and a half weeks, you would not survive outside of my womb and whatever was going to happen would happen. I was too early in my pregnancy for them to stop it. I would just have to sit at home and wait it out. I couldn't believe my ears! I was calling a doctor who was supposed to be there to help me, and he was now telling me he couldn't help. I could lose my precious long-awaited angel! I was given instructions to call if my water broke or if bleeding started, and to lie down and rest in the mean time.

I sobbed as I hung up the phone in defeat. I was so stunned that I couldn't even speak. It took your daddy about ten minutes to calm me before words could even come to my mouth. I was mortified by the details I had just been given. I couldn't believe that this was happening after all that we had been through to get you here. I finally was able to relay the grim news as your daddy settled me onto the couch and listened with a concerned ear.

Immediately we prayed. Then we called our family for prayer. And they called everyone and anyone they could think of to pray for your safety and protection. Then I made a distraught phone call to my place of work telling them I would be in touch and that I would let them know what was going on after being seen by a doctor the next day.

Your daddy was to speak at church that night, but wanted to stay at home with us to make sure all was going to be all right. Feeling a little more confident, I encouraged him to go and your Grammy came and sat with me until he returned home. While he was there, the church held us up in special prayer. I believe that helped get me through because the contractions defiantly persisted on, consistently coming every four to five minutes despite my rest. I contracted like that for eight terrifying hours. Finally, near midnight, they began to retreat and peace hovered over us. It appeared we would make it through the rest of the night.

Early the next morning, I called the doctor's office, filling the nurse in on the scary events that had taken place. She had us come into the office right away to be examined. The doctor found my cervix to be shortened and soft with a fingertip dilation. He also found an "abnormal" bulge down low where you had prematurely descended further into my pelvis. I was taken off work and placed on modified bed rest. I was to refrain from all contraction-causing activities such as walking and lifting.

It proved to be a very stressful week, spending every waking moment on the flat of my back not knowing what the outcome was going to be. I continued to be plagued by the contractions, and even was awakened out of sleep at night with hard menstrual-like cramps, which sent me fretfully to the phone calling the doctor again. I was told I could come and spend the night at the hospital until high-risk OB could see me or just wait at home until morning and be seen first thing. We chose the latter because of Hope and the fact that they really couldn't do anything for me once I was there.

The next morning we wearily went to be evaluated by the high-risk OB team at our hospital. I was found to have a positive fetal fibronectin, which indicates the likelihood of pre-term labor. I was given medication to keep pre-term labor at bay and was warily sent home to rest and to be on guard of my unstable pregnancy. I ended up in the doctor's office or the high-risk clinic every day that week. No one could figure out why this was happening and we were on the verge of exhaustion from the long nights and stress. We all prayed that God would keep His hand upon us and we praised Him for each passing day that I was still carrying you in the safety of my womb. Fortunately, we received an answer to our pleading prayers when subsequent fetal fibronectins came back negative and my cervix firmed up again.

It seems we are presently out of immediate danger, but I still need to be very cautious in everything I do. We go to the doctor for weekly exams to closely observe any new changes. I am so thankful that my doctors have an understanding of how priceless and valuable this pregnancy is, mainly because of how difficult it was to conceive and what we had to endure to get you here. They are not risking anything and are watching me very closely. I am so grateful for that.

God has given me peace now and I feel like things are going to be all right. I am hoping and praying that things will calm down very soon for us. Please hang in there, Jayden. I love you so much and I want you to remain safe so that you can grow healthy and strong. I am so sorry that this is happening to you. I believe God has His hand of protection on both of us and that He will hold you safely until it is time for you to come into this world. I love you with all of my heart and I don't want to lose you. I promise to be extremely careful in order to protect you and this pregnancy. I will do whatever it takes to keep you out of jeopardy, even if it means remaining on bed rest for the continuation of my pregnancy. Any sacrifice will be worth having you.

Trusting in the Lord,
Mommy

January 17, 2001

To my sweet bundle of joy,

Just a brief note to let you know that we looked at your heart today during our scheduled fetal echo. It seems that God has blessed you with a perfect heart and everything looks normal. Thank the Lord! That comes as a huge relief and much-needed good news after this past week of turmoil.

The technician inspected all four chambers of your heart and surrounding areas thoroughly and found no defects. We watched as you sprinted around in my belly. At one point, you did a "belly flop," turning your back to us. You seem to be quite the little gymnast in there! When you finally calmed down, you came to rest with your legs spread wide open like a frog. The technician pounced on the opportunity and printed a picture of your "pee-pee" for us! Don't worry; Mommy will keep it under wraps! I must confess, we proudly shared it with our family, doing away with any doubts that you are truly a boy.

I am still contracting on and off daily, but I am at peace about it. I have also been taken back off of my medication since my last fetal fibronectin was negative. That was a welcomed decision because the medicine gave me awful headaches. As frightening as it is, I am keeping my faith and trust in God that He will get us through this. I will be twenty-four weeks in a matter of days and you will be viable outside of my womb. We will be comforted when we meet that important milestone. Right now, I am centered on staying pregnant and spending time with you as I lay in bed. Because of all that has happened, I have been forced to bring my life to a halt and focus on you. We now spend special time together as I hold you in my tummy and rub and pat you. I love to talk to you and feel you move inside of me. Love floods over me every time we make a connection with each other. You are so very special to me.

With high hopes for our future,

Mommy

March 7, 2001

To my sweet angel baby boy,
Hello, dear baby. Our past few weeks have consisted mainly of resting in bed. I have been doing very little and going stir-crazy in the process. The highlights of my week are our doctor's visits and the occasional trip to church. That is only allowed if I have had a good day with minimal contractions, and once there, I must remain seated in the pew. I have had to leave early a few times because the contractions would creep up on me again, disrupting our outing.

My coworkers have sent me a wonderful surprise. They pitched in and made me a care basket. It was filled with goodies and projects to pamper myself and to help consume my time. It was so thoughtful of them and helpful, too.

It is getting very difficult because we are soon to be in the process of moving. I am unable to pack or prepare anything for our move at the end of the month to your grandparent's home. Thankfully, our parents, family members, and friends have pitched in and have been a great help. They have even started packing for us. They are helping to relieve a tremendous burden.

Poor Hope needs a mommy and I am trapped by these contractions, forcing me to prioritize between you and your sister. I know she would understand if she was old enough and she has really been a good sport through all of this. Your daddy has fallen under the load of the housework and managing a preschooler, but is patiently doing his best caring for all of us. I feel so guilty not being able to help more. Sometimes, if I am feeling well enough, I do get up and organize a few things, but quickly find myself retreating back to the bed or couch, conquered once again by the returning contractions. I know our hard work will pay off in the end and one day our lives will return to normal. Whatever that is!

We have celebrated another landmark in our pregnancy with you. I have met the twenty-eight week mark! You now have a 70% chance of survival outside of my womb. Keeping in mind the facts of our past rocky weeks, that comes as a huge relief and reassurance. God has been so good to us. I am taking in every moment I have with you during this pregnancy, knowing very well this is probably my one and only. I continue to thank God every day for this miracle I carry.

The time has already come for us to start our childbirth classes. I can't believe how time has flown by. I am excited to have a new adventure added to my usually ho-hum week. I was anxious for your daddy to attend these classes so he will have a fuller understanding of what to expect while I am in labor and delivering you. I am sure that I will learn a few things, too. I think that these classes add some reality to the fact that your impending arrival is near. It has felt like we are living in a dream (and occasionally a nightmare).

Our first class tonight went very well. We were one of ten couples attending the class. It is one of the largest classes they have had. It will last approximately five or six weeks, depending on how fast we move through the material. They gave us a nice book to refer to and some samples, along with parenting magazines to review. This first class covered the basics such as dilation, effacement and engagement. It was nothing that was foreign to me. However, I think your daddy learned a few new things. I am hoping that these classes prove beneficial to us as we labor for you.

I have been thinking a lot about my labor and delivery. At times I am gripped by fear, so I have come to a decision. Anytime a negative thought regarding your delivery tries to gain access to my mind, I immediately chase them away with positive ones. After all, millions of women have given birth before me and lived to tell about it. So I can, too! I am strong and determined and I know God won't put more on me than I can bear. I can do it! I intend on focusing on these things as I am challenged by my labor pains. I know that I can do all things through Christ who strengthens me. I can do it! Besides, these pains will be a good thing. They will be bringing you to me. We have already withstood so much, I am sure I can tolerate a little more in order to have you, my sweet desire. I will let you know if this plan works or not.

Well, my love, rest well and continue to grow healthy and strong. I pray daily for your health and protection so that we make it to term. Every passing day is an answered prayer. God has been faithful to us. I love you, my angel!

Patiently waiting,
Mommy

March 14, 2001

To my precious angel,

Jayden, time is passing by so quickly! We have nine weeks or less until we meet. It feels like I blinked, then—here we are. I am so anxious to finally have you in my arms, yet I want more time to get things prepared for you. It wouldn't be so bad if our new home was complete and I could assemble your nursery. We are set to move out of our current home at the end of the month and move in with your daddy's parents temporarily. Our home is due to be complete in May or June. I have a strong feeling that you will be here before our home will.

I have been preparing for you the best that I can. I told you how I had your crib picked out years before you were even conceived and then how we fell upon the very last one. Your great-grandfather, Pap Battisti, wanted to purchase it for you instead, along with the white bedding set that was displayed inside of the crib. He also bought us a white-spindled changing table that matches the crib nicely. Your grandmother Donham, Me-maw, wants to purchase a white gliding rocker for our baby shower. I am looking forward to that as we cuddle together. So far, the only large item your daddy and I have had to purchase was a beautiful white glossy chest of drawers with white ceramic and brass handles decorating the front. Best of all, we got it on clearance and only had to pay eight-seven dollars of the original two hundred and seventeen-dollar price tag! That was truly a blessing for us. We hope to get most of the remaining necessities at our baby showers.

Being confined on modified bed rest, I did a lot of research on the

Internet as to how we would decorate your new nursery. We have chosen the pattern "Serendipity" by Kid's Line. It is a whimsical Noah's ark pattern in rich blues and golden yellow stars decorated with colorful funny animals. I thought it was adorable. And when I found out that it came in round bedding, I was ecstatic! I knew I had to have it for you. I went on a bit of a scavenger hunt by phone, but luckily ran across it at a retail store in Pittsburgh. It was now a clearance item, since the bed was discontinued, and we got it for a wonderfully discounted price! I think it will be perfect for you, Jayden. We are hoping that your Poppy will be able to do a matching mural on the wall to fill your room with even more color and love.

I am glad I have been off work, although for reasons I would have preferred to never encounter. It has given me the opportunity to drink in every moment of this miraculous pregnancy. I will truly miss being pregnant. I try to enjoy and hold on to each new thing as we move quickly toward our due date. I realize this may be the last time I get to experience all of this. I am so thankful to have you, dear Jayden.

You are now extremely active in my belly. Sometimes you even wake me up during the night as you wriggle and roll around trying to get comfortable in my increasingly crowded abdomen. One of my favorite things to do now is to lie down while you are awake and lift my shirt up and watch my animated tummy as you dance all over the place. I can see just about every roll, kick and punch you give me. Sometimes it feels like you are going to spring right out of there! You are getting very big, too. That fact makes every move even more noticeable. It is especially odd when you turn to my right side, watching this alien-like object move and shift about until it wads up, creating a huge deformity in my stature. It is not very comfortable for either one of us and thankfully you do not stay in that position for very long. Your movements still bring wide smiles to my face. It is the most amazing and wonderful thing I have ever experienced in my life. I think it is even more special to me because this is something that I was not supposed to have. I was told that I would never become pregnant under our circumstances and now here you are! My miracle!

Well, sweet child, I am dreaming the days away with thoughts of you in my arms. It won't be long now until you are born, turning our world amazingly upside down with your love. I am watching the calendar for our due date and praying for you daily as you continue to grow and mature in my womb.

With all of my love,
Mommy

April 10, 2001

To my dear Jayden,

Sweet baby boy, you are growing larger and larger in my tight belly. My weight is toppling the scales as I continue to gain weekly. I am so happy you are growing perfectly strong while your lungs mature in my womb. You will be ready to come into this world very soon. We have just six short weeks or less!

I have continued to contract as always. Fortunately, my cervix is not changing, but I continue to be examined every week just to be safe. I had some spotting and bleeding two weeks ago that was alarming, but it quit as swiftly as it began. Thank the Lord!

Another side effect of this pregnancy is swelling. I woke up on April 5th with enormous legs. I couldn't find my ankles and I had pitting edema from my thighs to my feet. I could make a deep indentation in my extremities when I depressed a finger into them. My blood pressure and urine checked out OK, so it is just another thing to keep a watch on. I can't squeeze into my shoes and I can't get my wedding band off my stubby finger. I have graduated to ugly clog-style shoes for the time being. Between my excess weight and the newly acquired edema, I really have a waddle going on when I walk!

Speaking of walking, another contributor to my "waddle" is the fact that my joints are loosening up from the normal hormonal changes in my body. This is in preparation for your birth, so my bones will separate and make room for your head to pass through. Because of this phenomenon, I snap, crackle, and pop like the cereal. It makes my walking much different and turning over in bed almost impossible. I literally have to place my hands under my hips to turn my pelvis, as it cracks and pops during the turn. Then I aid my big belly the same way until we are all facing in the same direction. It can get quite uncomfortable, but it is all for you to get here.

On Saturday, April 4th, we had our baby shower. When I arrived at the church I was overwhelmed. I had never seen such a gorgeous baby shower in all of my life. And it was packed full of surprises.

As I entered the doorway, I passed through several tall white columns. They were adorned with flowing baby blue netting marking the entrance to this grand celebration. Stationed at different areas in the room were beautiful tables decorated with white linen table clothes and skirted with white lights and baby blue netting. They overflowed with delicacies and delicious hors d'oeuvres. One table housed an ornate silver fountain with red punch cascading down on pillow tops of sherbet. At the main table, salads were served on china with my favorite "Olive Garden" salad dressing. Also at that table were soft blue napkins with a sweet little angel and the words, "Welcome angel baby, Jayden Bryan" embossed on the center. In the front of the room was a table for me, the guest of honor, my mom, and my mother-in-law. Our table and all of the guest tables were garnished with creative centerpieces that were actually gifts for us! Each one was different and uniquely decorated. They were so adorable. Front and center was set up for me with a white wicker rocker and a stork announcing, "It's a boy" from its beak. To the right of my rocking chair was the gift table spilling over with an abundance of baby gifts for you.

I couldn't believe it! Everything was exquisite and perfect. I couldn't get over how much effort my friends and sister-in-law put into this event. And it was all to celebrate you!

We had a marvelous time as my friend, Christy, welcomed our guests, reminiscing my difficult time of infertility and how we have been miraculously blessed by your impending arrival. Your Grammy said a special prayer for us and blessed the food. Afterward, your Me-maw spoke and referred to scripture in the Bible. It was all very touching. I was then placed up front in the wicker rocking chair to start my way through the mound of gifts that were waiting for me. Hope and her friend Makenzie joined in making the gift opening a bit of a relay race. We received many beautiful and useful things that we needed. I was so appreciative of everyone's generosity toward us. I gave the biggest heartfelt thank you that I could and then said goodbye and passed out hugs and kisses to our guests. It was an amazing day.

It took several cars to load up your new belongings to take back to your grandparent's house, where we are now temporarily residing. Once there, we were able to separate and sort through everything. We took a closer look at the things we barely got to glance at in the midst of the excitement at the shower. As I looked over the tiny baby clothes, diapers and cute baby toys, I began to ponder what it was going to be like having you here using these things. It almost didn't seem real to me.

Today we had a second baby shower given by my coworkers at the cancer center. I made my way to the conference room this afternoon and propped my swollen feet up on chairs as they served cake and ice cream to my attentive guests. I had not been able to see them for weeks and everyone was amazed at the weight I had put on and at my now very large and prominent abdomen. Everyone wanted to touch and rub my large belly, feeling you packed tightly inside. We were welcomed there by a bountiful pile of gifts, too. I didn't get one duplicate gift. Everything was just what we needed and appreciated very much.

Now we are all set for you, sweet baby. In a matter of weeks our fantasy will be over and we will be holding our dream. I am now on the brink of the moment I have waited for my whole life. Things have been surreal. I continue to enjoy these last moments with you in my tummy and I fear these contractions less and less. I will see you soon, my angel!

With great expectations,

Mommy

May 3, 2001

To my precious Jayden,

Today marks a very sad day in our lives, sweet child. Your cousin Ashley has gone to be with the Lord today. After battling congenital heart disease for her thirteen precious years of life, she fought a brave last fight from complications of a staph infection and congestive heart failure. It was more than her frail heart could endure. Now the family joins together as they try to pick up the pieces to their broken hearts from this tragedy. Our loss has been heaven's gain as we say goodbye to this sweet angel.

The past weeks have been filled with frantic phone calls, desperate prayers, and emotional pleas during Ashley's struggle in the intensive care unit. This recent illness came unexpectedly. Her condition had been stable over the past few years. Your grandparents have been traveling back and forth to Virginia and North Carolina to comfort their son and first-born granddaughter. Now they mourn for her and pull together to support their son in their tragic heartbreak. They have felt pulled between their grief and the impending arrival of their grandson. I assured them that it was OK to be there for Jerry and Ashley and not to worry about us. If I were to give birth to you while they were gone, they would still have the rest of their lives to be with you. If it were not for my near due date and complications I have already suffered, we would be there to support the family also.

There have been some slight changes for us. In my 35th week, I had a lot of gastrointestinal upset. So bad in fact, I actually lost a little weight at that week's doctor's visit. I felt then that it was a precursor to your arrival. I have been doing some serious contracting since that point, too. I got into a good pattern a couple of times and thought I was on my way to the hospital. Just as I would prepare to go, things would calm down again. That week I was found to be one to two centimeters dilated, 70% effaced, and -2 station. After all of these weeks of contracting and no changes in my cervix, this was welcome news, even though a little early. I don't want you to come too soon, but I was ready to see some progress.

At today's appointment I was two to three centimeters dilated and still 70% effaced and at -2 station. My doctor decided to strip my membranes to possibly encourage things along a bit now that I am 38 weeks. I am so happy that we have made it to term. You can come anytime now and it will be safe for you. I have our bags packed for the hospital and ready to go on the spur of the moment, if necessary. We have set a date for induction if you don't come before hand. We will go into the hospital on the evening of the 10th and you should be born on May 11th. Isn't it ironic how we have tried desperately not to go into premature labor all of this time, and now that we have reached full term, we may need to have an induction? The nurse reassures us that this is typical. I guess we are now on the final countdown.

Anxiously counting the days,

Mommy

May 10, 2001

To my sweet Jayden Bryan,

Welcome to the world, my precious miracle baby! My dream has come true! Today I hold you in my arms. This has been the most spectacular event of my life! I am humbled by the awesome power and healing wonders of God.

On May 4th, I had a lot of contractions and also lost my mucous plug. Your daddy's parents went to Virginia to be with your Uncle Jerry after the death of Ashley. Things had been a bit chaotic with the recent events. Family came and went. The telephone rang endlessly as a multitude of phone calls poured in from well-wishers paying their respects for Ashley's passing.

That evening, we decided to go out to dinner. I noticed my contractions had picked up and were coming rather rhythmically. I was becoming quite uncomfortable during our dinner and I announced to your daddy that I thought this would be "the night." On our way home, we bumped into your daddy's sister, Aunt Dee, and her family on their way to Virginia. We excitedly gave them the news and said we would be in touch from the hospital. We went home to get things in order and to time the contractions a little closer. I did some laundry that was piling and the dishes. Then I pulled out the pre-packed suitcases and began to get Hope ready to stay with your Aunt Barbara. That's when I noticed that the contractions had slowed down considerably. The discomfort that I previously had in my back was now invisible and the contractions that were left were spacing further and further apart. My labor had stopped. We called our families and told them it was a false alarm, but we would keep them posted.

A few days later, your grandparents returned home and we continued on with the sporadic labor patterns starting and stopping. On May 7th, I had a doctor's appointment that measured me at three centimeters, 70% effaced and -2 station. It looked like the induction was on for the evening of May 10th, but at least I had a good running start.

Your grandparents and most of your daddy's family were leaving again for a final memorial service for Ashley on May 9th.They would leave Virginia the next day and be home in time for my induction so they wouldn't miss your arrival. Before they left, Your Pap-Pap placed his hand on my tummy and prayed that if you were to be born before they got home, the delivery would be safe, quick and painless. We hugged and wished them a safe trip. I told them I would wait for them to come home, but if something happened before they got back, not to rush. We would be waiting on them in the hospital.

I didn't feel well the day of the 9th. Between all that had happened with Ashley, the stress on the family, us not being moved into our new home yet, and all of the normal fatigues of late pregnancy (such as waking eight times in the night to pee), I had an uncomfortable backache and we decided not to go to church. My back pains got worse so I decided to get on my hands and knees to help ease some of the pressure of the huge load I was carrying. Up to this point I had gained fifty-five pounds! This was not doing the trick as my discomfort grew, so I decided to go stand in the shower. Warm water pelted over my aching back, giving it some relief. I started to shower and shave my legs, but I was so tired and miserable. I decided to just stand there and be lazy. I figured I would worry about it the next day before I went to the hospital.

I wearily retreated to bed where I struggled to drift off to sleep. I finally found some solace and was able to get a little rest. Just as I was drifting off into a deep slumber, a hard pain hit my back and surged around my abdomen. Hard cramping consumed me. I shot up in bed, groaning, as I realized my irritable bowel syndrome must have been flaring up. Glancing over at the clock I noticed it was now 11:30 at night. I miserably made my way to the bathroom when—bam! There it was again. I ran for the restroom this time, because my stomach was now terribly upset. To my surprise, I was not obtaining relief and my back pain was accompanied by contractions. Now my mind raced as I thought, *Wait a minute—I think I am in labor.* Boom! Another one hit. I hobbled to the bedroom where your daddy was just getting settled into the warm cozy blankets.

"Don't get too comfortable," I warned. "We are going to the hospital tonight!" He whined something back at me about not having any rest, so I gave him permission to lie in bed until I showered and shaved my legs (unshaved legs is every pregnant woman's nightmare).

I made my way back to the bathroom in discomfort. My contractions were spaced four or five minutes apart, but as soon as I got into the shower I noticed them coming more rapidly, about every two to three minutes. Now they had great intensity. Not caring that I was a guest in someone's home anymore, I flung the shower door open with water spraying everywhere. I propped my swollen legs up on the brass cushioned vanity seat to easily shave them. All the while I was struggling against the intense shooting pain that was increasingly getting worse. It continued to travel from my back to my lower abdomen. When a contraction came, I had to stop what I was doing just to get through it. As my pain intensified, I remembered my previous plan. I was going to do this!

When my contraction started, I would begin "talking down" to it. I would repeat things like, "I can do it! I can do it! Dear Lord, this really, really hurts, but I can do it! I know I can do this!" I was moaning some in between, but it really helped when I took control and told my contraction who was boss. As the pains got harder, my voice got louder. Your daddy heard the argument between me and my contraction. Not sure who was winning, he flung the door open and asked if I was OK. I think he was just getting the picture that I was serious when I said I was in labor. It takes your poor daddy a little time to catch on.

At that point the contractions were coming about every two minutes and stronger than ever. That meant I only had one precious pain-free minute at a time to get anything accomplished. I frantically scurried around trying to get ready. I ordered your daddy to get the bags in the car, run Hope across the yard to his Aunt Barbara, and to get me clothes—any clothes, whether they matched or not. It wasn't important now. I was ready to go to the hospital in my towel! There was no time to worry about making a fashion statement.

I finally managed to get myself dressed and I pulled my dripping wet hair back into a combed hair band. My original plans of looking like a Barbie doll went flying out the window as my pain took precedence. I continued pep talking myself through the contractions as I slowly made my way to the car, pausing for the contractions.

As we were driving to the hospital in the wee hours of the morning, I sensed your daddy's nervousness. He gripped my hand as I verbalized to my contractions that they hurt, they hurt really badly, but I was strong and I could do it. A couple of times my mind drifted off and a contraction unexpectedly crept up on me. I thought I would lose control. I learned my lesson quickly that in order to get through these painful contractions, I would have to stay on top of them and keep reminding myself that I was in charge and I could handle it.

My thoughts went back to Ashley and your daddy's family. They were going to miss your birth after all. They had been going through one of the most terrible events of their life, and now they were going to miss out on one of the happiest.

Oddly enough, history seemed to be repeating itself. Thirteen years ago when Ashley was born, her heart condition came as a shock to her unsuspecting family. Not knowing whether she was going to live or die, the family was called to Virginia as Ashley lay helplessly in the neonatal intensive care unit with her seriously malformed heart struggling to beat on. Your daddy's parents arrived and immediately were captivated by their firstborn grandchild. They were crushed as they saw her in such a fragile condition. While in Virginia with their son, his wife, and little Ashley, they received a call from home in West Virginia. It was their daughter Shelly, who was also expecting. She was in labor and she was scared. She wanted her parents with her. Torn between their ailing granddaughter and their laboring daughter in Morgantown, they finally decided to head home for the delivery after Ashley stabilized.

Shortly after their arrival, Gregory "Adam" Cummings made his. There was such drama surrounding Ashley's birth as she and her cousin Adam caused everyone to move frantically from one hospital to the other. Now we faced a similar scenario in her death.

As another contraction jolted my thoughts back to my labor, I realized we were still in the car. I ordered your daddy to drive faster and get us to the hospital before you made an unwanted appearance in the car. We were coming upon a stoplight that had just turned red, so I warned him to not even think about stopping. There was no traffic and if a cop spotted us, I was sure he would understand. My priority was to get to the hospital, especially before I lost my window of opportunity to receive an epidural (the epidural was high on my priority list). I was able to tolerate the pain, but I wasn't sure how bad it was going to get and I didn't want to risk not being able to have something for comfort.

After a grueling ride that seemed to last forever, we finally made it to the emergency room. My contractions were one on top of the other and I couldn't walk. I sent your daddy to get help for me. A nurse bolted out of the emergency room door in a frenzy yelling, "Do you feel the urge to push?"

I replied, "No, but I feel the urge for an epidural!" At least I hadn't lost my sense of humor yet. They eased me into a wheelchair and parked me at the registration desk. I was beginning to wonder what I was doing wrong that no one had got the picture yet. I was in labor! I needed to be in the delivery room—not the registration room! I breathlessly mumbled my information to the clerk as I continued to tackle my contractions with my positive thinking strategy. It kind of sounded like, "Yes, my name is Dorothy—(Deep breath) I can do this—It really hurts—I know I can do it—I am going to make it—(Panting)—(Blowing)—Donham and I am in labor." I guess I should have told the nurse I had the urge to push so that I would have received a prompt ride to labor and delivery, skipping the fiasco in registration.

I was finally whisked away in my wheelchair, stopping for contractions by my ever-so-patient escort. I was wheeled briskly to the triage room with wet hair blowing in the wind. My escort did comment on how good my hair smelled. I was glad to know that not all of my attempts at primping went in vain!

I looked up at the clock as I was being helped onto the exam table and noted that it was now 1:30 a.m. A helpful nurse introduced herself as she got me situated and began taking some of my medical history. A short time later, a resident arrived to examine me and found that I was six centimeters dilated, 90% effaced, and at zero station. I was definitely staying until you would be delivered.

After my exam, I continued to have one contraction after the next. With one of my harder contractions I felt a "pop" and then a warm gush of fluid as my bag of water broke. I notified the nurse and she checked the fluid. When I moved off of my pad, we noted a slimy green fluid and she confirmed that indeed my water had broken. She placed me on the monitor and left the room to inform the doctor. Too caught up in my contractions, I hadn't given the sight a second thought. The pain was so intense, nausea overwhelmed me and I began to dry heave uncontrollably until some of the nausea subsided.

Since I was definitely in labor and I was dilated to six centimeters, we decided to call my parents and your daddy's sister Aunt Dee. She was the only family member on your daddy's side who lived in town and had not gone to Ashley's memorial service. That was at 2:30 a.m.

I was moved to the labor and delivery room and settled into the bed. I had to have an IV started, blood work drawn, and IV fluid infused before I could get an epidural, because they are notorious for causing low blood pressure. My mom arrived at 3:00 a.m. shortly before I could get my epidural. She was ecstatic that the day had finally come for us, even if it was in the middle of the night. My contractions continued to intensify and I would grip the bed rails and moan with them, sometimes loudly to get through it. Afterward, I would apologize for any noise I had made. I was quickly reassured that I was fine and doing a great job. I didn't realize how important and beneficial that encouragement would be until I was actually in labor.

My nurse offered me Phenergan for the nausea and Nubain to hold me over until I could have an epidural. When one is in the position I was, it was an offer hard to refuse. Now looking in hindsight, I wished that I would not have taken it because I didn't have any more nausea and it didn't help my pain. It only made me feel loopy and drugged. I literally couldn't hold my eyes open, even though I felt wide-awake. I could only peek out of one eye when someone talked to me. My nurse continued to be very attentive to my needs. So much so, I told her in my medicated stupor that she was the most wonderful nurse I ever had. And in a very grateful tone I announced that if our baby turned out to be a girl, I would name it after her. She laughed and thanked me diplomatically.

My contractions continued to come frequently and I continued to "positive think" my way through them. That seemed to help me. I couldn't believe how my plan was actually working. A couple of times the contractions were fierce and came furiously as pain wracked over my back and abdomen. I held the side rails so tightly I thought I would rip them off the bed. My nurse would step in and remind me to do my breathing exercises, help me to gain control once again, and congratulate me on doing such a good job. It truly gave me the confidence that I needed to handle the next one. I was surprised to find that fear was more of the aggravator than the pain.

At one point, Mom was on the phone with Dad giving him an update. She whispered in the phone that I was in a lot of pain and was crying (which I was not). Mom always tends to get caught up in a situation when giving details. Wanting Dad to know that I was not that bad off, I turned over in bed, opened my eyes wide, and said in my everyday voice, "I am not crying, I am just moaning—It helps me get through my contraction. I am doing just fine." With that she shrugged her shoulders and told Dad I was fine. I was not about to give in to my labor. I was going to work with it instead.

Around 3:30 a.m. I received my long-awaited epidural. I lay hunched over the bedside table in your daddy's arms while the anesthesiologist placed the catheter in my spine. I flinched from the needle prick, but shortly after I started to receive the relief I was waiting for as the medication flowed through my pain-stricken body. As he was taping the dressing up my back, your Aunt Dee arrived. I informed the anesthesiologist that I loved him and that he was the most wonderful doctor there. Another lesson learned: make a laboring woman happy—she will be your friend for life!

The anesthesiologist was just as attentive as my nurse, checking on me frequently, making sure my pain was under control, and ensuring that I was as pain-free as possible. I did have a "window" in my abdomen that wouldn't numb, so I continued to experience my contractions for a few hours as he continued to bolus me with pain medication trying to catch up to my pain. He was honestly a very good doctor. I am sure both he and my nurse were quite amused by the love and admiration I now had for the both of them as they worked to make me comfortable.

Aunt Dee stayed by my side along with my mom and your daddy, helping me to get through the contractions. I didn't realize how parched my mouth was from all of the groaning until your Aunt Dee offered me ice chips. Never in my life had I noticed how wonderful ice chips tasted until that night. I was too tired by this point to verbalize to my contractions anymore, so I just breathed through them. Mom laughed at me because after moaning noisily with a contraction, I would perk up and say, "That wasn't so bad!" Becoming exhausted with the pain and thoroughly enjoying my minute of rest between contractions, I cringed and sighed in defeat, "Oh no, another one is coming already!" I changed positions several times trying to get the epidural to take affect to that stubborn painful area in my abdomen to no avail.

Shortly after the epidural, the resident came back to check my cervix and said that I had already progressed to a whopping nine centimeters! It was all moving so fast. It seemed like I had just checked in. He also informed me that when my water had broken, they confirmed that it was stained with meconium. That explained the slimy green matter in the fluid I had seen earlier, but had allowed it to simply pass through my mind. I was certainly attentive now, knowing the risk this carried for you. You had your first bowel movement in utero and this presented a certain danger for you. If you happen to swallow any of it, you could aspirate it into your lungs and develop pneumonia or an infection, both of which could cause you to be placed on a ventilator. That could lead to many more risks and complications, even death. He assured me that they would be prepared at the time of your birth by having pediatricians present to examine you as soon as you were born. He also warned me that because of this complication, I would not be able to hold you right away. Instead, they would pass you directly to the waiting pediatric team to immediately check your lungs. Even though that was disappointing, my thoughts and heart were focused on you and your safety. Whatever we had to do to ensure your health was all that I was concerned with.

About an hour later, the nurse found that I was now complete. I had reached a full ten centimeters in a matter of about five hours and could start pushing as soon as I felt the urge to do so. With my epidural now taking full effect, I was able to fully relax and feel pain-free. Being without pain allowed the exhaustion and fatigue to consume me. Your head was still up high so the nurse decided to let me rest and allow the contractions to pull you down some before we started to push. I quickly fell asleep, occasionally being awakened by my own snoring. To my dismay, I caught your daddy with a video camera in my face as unmentionable sounds escaped my nose. I would jolt awake self-consciously from the loud snorts only to find everyone hovering around my bed staring at me. Someone would rub my head and encourage me to get my rest and I would again slip back into my slumber until the next rumble awakened me.

After an hour or so of rest and still no urge to push, we all made a joint decision to get the ball rolling. The nurse sat the squat bar up on the bed for me to hold on to while I balanced myself in a crouched position on the mattress. This was to let gravity play a role in helping us out. Deanna watched the monitor and told me when I was having a contraction so I could push. She counted to ten, and I pushed at least three times within the one contraction. I pushed with all of my might, hoping to bring your head down for delivery. Your daddy lay sleeping in the recliner, wiped out from the night's exciting but exhausting events. Your grammy took pictures in amusement while I pushed. She was fascinated by how many shades of red and purple my face turned as I attempted to force you out.

She said in amazement, "Dorothy, your face is turning so purple!"

I thought, *I am trying to give birth to something the size of a watermelon, and you can't believe my face is purple?* We all laughed as I continued to work. After about an hour or more of pushing we found that nothing was happening and the nurse told me to take another break because your heart rate was consistently remaining in the 180s, causing alarm considering the previous complication of meconium that we were already aware of. After some rest, my contractions picked up, but your heart rate didn't slow down.

It was time to call the doctor in. She quickly arrived and assessed the situation as I apologized to my poor nurse for what was going to be a change of shift baby. Having worked in the hospital myself, I knew that all the drama seems to occur at the change of shift. My doctor came over to my bedside to tell me the plan. We had to get you out and we had to do it quickly. Your heart rate was up, you were in apparent distress and we couldn't play around. My heart sank as her words unraveled in my hazy mind.

"Does this mean I have to have a cesarean section?" I fretfully asked. She said not yet, and that we would try to get you out with a vacuum-assisted delivery. I agreed. It was time to get down to business.

Pictures on the wall swung open, closets unfolded, and bright lights came down from the ceiling as they sat up the room around me with equipment preparing for the imminent delivery. People filled the room as a pediatric team arrived to take care of any possible complications you could have. Extra nurses came in to be on hand to help with my delivery and baby nurses stood at the infant warmer waiting for you. Fear of the pain I would feel during your delivery plagued my mind. I made it through labor OK, but what was this going to be like? How well was my epidural working now? Would I still feel pain through it? I quickly chased those thoughts out of my head with thoughts of your sweet face I was about to meet. I was positioned in the stirrups with your Aunt Dee on one side and my nurse on the other. I motioned for your daddy to grab the video camera for Aunt Dee and to come help support me, but in the organized chaos of the now busy room, he grabbed the camera and started snapping pictures along with your Grammy.

The nurse and Aunt Dee supported my back to help me curl over my bulging belly. They also helped me to hold my legs back, opening my pelvis for your delivery. My doctor instructed me to push with everything in me because we had to get you out. With the next contraction, I drew a deep breath and plunged every ounce of strength I had toward pushing you out to safety. Just as I started to lose my stamina, they coached me and persuaded me to push even harder before taking my next deep breath. My eyes were scrunched shut as I used every muscle in my body to push with. Your head was starting to crown and the vacuum was applied to your scalp.

I heard Aunt Dee's voice break while she was counting. Emotions poured over her and also filled the room. *Thank you, God*, I thought. *Thank you for my miracle. My angel baby is coming—he is coming!* Those thoughts gave me even more power and determination to push you out.

Everyone cheered as your head started to make its way out. While I was pushing, I curled up even further around my belly to see what was going on. As I leaned over, I saw your precious head making its descent into the world. At that moment it all became real to me. It was no longer a dream—you were a reality. I became so emotional I lost my breath that I was pushing with while tears of joy erupted from my soul. I quickly had to compose myself and gasp a new breath, because the priority was still to deliver you quickly.

After your head was delivered, I lay back on the bed to gain more strength while the doctor deep suctioned your airway. She was attempting to remove any possible meconium before you drew your first breath. As she was doing so, she cautioned us not to be alarmed. We would hopefully not hear you cry right away. They wanted to get a quick look into your lungs before you were able to aspirate anything into them.

I felt the presence of God in there with us giving us all strength and peace as I continued to deliver you. Just minutes after your head was out, the rest of you quickly followed. I watched in amazement as your precious life was pulled from mine. It was truly a defining moment in my life. It was the most spectacular thing I had ever witnessed! I couldn't believe this was happening to me and I was finally laying eyes on my angel baby that took so many years, so much heartache, and an abundance of tears to get here. I felt like I was the first woman who had ever given birth. I felt so triumphant at that moment—like an Olympian being awarded the gold medal.

On May 10, 2001, at 8:27 a.m., my unanswered prayer became my miracle. My angel baby was born!

I watched nervously as the doctor handed your limp body over to the waiting pediatric team. They intubated you, placing a laryngoscope into your airway, inspecting your lungs and suctioning you out in the process. The room became uncomfortably silent.

My doctor said, "I told you he wasn't going to cry right away."

I desperately peered from my bed, trying to see through the crowd of medical personnel working on you, watching their every move. Your daddy grabbed the video camera and made his way through the staff to record your first minutes of life. Moments later, you gave a glorious loud newborn cry that broke the dreaded silence. The whole room erupted as relief replaced fear. Tears were shed, but I was still too worried to even cry—I needed to see my baby.

The nurses reported to me from across the room how big you were and how much dark hair covered your head. That especially surprised us because both of our families come from a long line of bald, eventually blond babies. I remembered the secret prayers I whispered during my pregnancy, praying that God would give you just a little bit of hair and not let you be "shiny bald." How my prayers were once again answered. I could see that every inch of your head was covered in dark hair. We were stunned. The nurse placed a hat on your head and wrapped you tightly in warm blankets. My heart pounded as she made her way toward me with my angel in her arms. With my arms all ready outstretched toward you, she made her way across the room to my side, placing my long-awaited miracle from heaven in my arms at last. I was so overwhelmed and consumed by emotion, that tears still could not come. My emotional state was beyond tears. All that could escape me was whimpers of astonishment. I held you so tightly and so close. It was as if time stood still and we were the only two people in the room. I blocked out all of the noise and busyness around me, even the doctors who were still working on me. It was just my angel and me—like long lost loves from the past once again reunited. The most eloquent, descriptive words could not begin to describe the way I felt at that moment. A tidal wave of love washed over me for you and for those first precious moments, we basked in it together.

I looked up to your daddy, who had been leaning over us, and proudly said, "I told you I could do it!" We all laughed as I reveled in my victory. Now, caught up in the moment, I said, "Here, hold your son," as I handed you over to him. He wept as the same feelings I had experienced now flooded over him. After we counted your fingers and toes, your Aunt Dee and Grammy got their turn to cuddle you, too. I wish that I could relate to you the joy and happiness you brought into our lives.

The nurse took you to obtain your weight and measure you. You weighed in at a scale-bending nine pounds and twelve and a half ounces! I knew you were going to be big, but I was not thinking ten pounds of big! You were twenty-one inches long and given a clean bill of health, perfect in every way. You were the most beautiful newborn I had ever laid eyes on! You looked almost exactly like my baby pictures, except you had your daddy's sharp, turned-up chin. Your head was covered in dark, matted hair. Your skin was smooth and milky. It was as soft as velvet. You were adorably plump all over. Your face was still a little swollen, but you definitely had those chubby cheeks we were expecting. We had kissed them so much already, I feared they would chap. You had the usual newborn deep blue-gray eyes that seemed to pierce right through our soul when you looked at us. Could it be that you truly realized how long it took us to get you here and just how special you really are?

You were returned back to my longing arms as I made my first attempts to breast feed you. As if we had been doing it forever, you nuzzled close to me and nursed without any difficulty whatsoever. What a special time that was as I held you close and fed you. Our bonds deepened as we shared this intimate time together.

Your daddy made phone calls to our anxious family, who were anticipating this good news. He called his parents' cell phone in Virginia. They had no idea up to that point that I had even gone into labor, let alone you being here already. With you crying loudly in the background, he made the wonderful announcement that you had safely arrived. It was the news they needed after attending the memorial for Ashley, who had passed away just seven days earlier. The scripture came to their hearts, "Weeping endures for a night; but joy cometh in the morning." But in our case it was joy that cometh in the "mourning." The arrival of their seventh grandson was just what they needed. God was certainly faithful and full of mercy. We told them we would be waiting for them as they made their way to the hospital to meet you for the first time.

Your Grammy was also making phone calls just minutes after your birth to let our family know you were here and that everything was OK. She called Pap Battisti and let him hear you cry through the telephone. He was overjoyed! She also called your Poppy. He asked how everything went and she filled him in. She asked him if he would like to speak with me.

A little bewildered, he asked, "Is she well enough to talk?" He was sure I had been through a great ordeal and didn't think I would now have the strength to speak over the phone. Mom assured him I was fine and handed me the phone.

In an excited voice I answered, "Hello, Dad!" I proudly exclaimed that you had made it safely and that the birth was pain-free, which relieved my fears. I then announced that I could do this again! I would love to have the ability to give birth to another child. Dad was now thrilled, not only that his grandson had made it safely into the world, but that his daughter was not suffering. Instead, I was bubbling over with happiness. He told me that he would have to see us after work, but would be counting the minutes until then.

It wasn't even an hour later that he bounced through the door with his mom (Nanny) alongside of him. He was absolutely glowing as he took his first look at you. He proclaimed that he had waited nearly thirty years for this boy. Once he confirmed that I really was OK, he scooped you up into his anxious arms and fell deeply in love with you. Everyone in the room beamed. Nanny also got to hold you tightly as she made over all of your wonderful features. It is a miracle just seeing what one tiny little baby has brought into a whole family's life. We all experienced such a heightened sense of love today and thankfulness for my easy delivery and your good health.

Your Aunt Kathy rushed over from work with a friend. She also couldn't stand to wait until the end of her work day to meet her new nephew, whom she affectionately refers to as "precious." Your Great-grandma Ruby and Aunt Jan came shortly after your birth also. Our angel baby had finally arrived and so many people were excited to finally meet you.

Hope was finally brought in to meet her new baby brother. She was captivated by this new being that had been tucked away in Mommy's belly. Hope was thrilled to hold you and touch your soft head. We were touched by her gentle interaction with you as we watched a new bond develop between our children.

After the initial adrenalin rush we all experienced, the tired feelings soon overtook us after such a long but productive night. Your Aunt Dee went to work (I'll never know how she did it) and Grammy went home to sleep a little and to take care of herself because she is diabetic. Everyone else had to go back to work and about their day, once more leaving just you, your daddy, and me alone.

The nurse was now focused on my recovery, obtaining a breakfast tray and encouraging me to eat. Right after your birth I was so thirsty I downed a whole pitcher of ice water and asked for a refill. Now I had to find room for food to give my body the nourishment it needed to allow the process of milk production to begin. A little later on, the nurse attempted to set me up in the bed, preparing me for that first walk to the restroom. The room literally spun around me and a loud humming filled my ears as I warned I was about to pass out. My blood pressure had quickly dropped and I was in desperate need of intravenous fluids. I had lost a great deal of blood during delivery and my hemoglobin was low, contributing to my dizziness. After several bags of IV fluid, my blood pressure started to rise and I weakly, but successfully, made my first trip to the bathroom without incident. Afterward, we were transferred to a private patient room.

Although still very worn out, we hosted many other guests that came to see you on your birthday. That evening your Me-maw and Pap-Pap Donham finally arrived from Virginia to meet their newest grandchild. You brought such healing to their hurting hearts. Your head full of dark silky hair and your flawless chubby face took them aback. You looked so serene and contented. Instantly their hearts grew to hold love for yet another grandchild in their life.

This day has been incredible, my love. I hold you and gaze into your angelic face, wondering if you remember heaven and if maybe you did get to meet your Grandpa Musick. I certainly know that you were hand-picked by God. You are so special, sweet Jayden. You're an indescribable gift. What an extraordinary journey we have made to be together. I thought my life had come to an abrupt, unfortunate end as I felt my sanity slipping away from the empty arms I carried. They longed desperately to hold you, angel. Now I hold nearly all ten pounds of you in my arms that are wrapped tightly, contented and satisfied around your soft cuddly body. The arms of my heart that felt so empty and lonely have reached out and grabbed hold of you also. They will never let you go.

With a heart overflowing with love,

Mommy

Epilogue

I am amazed at how Jayden has made such an impact in our lives. The moment he was born, I learned how to love in a different way. I could have never fathomed the depth of that love. It immediately changed my perspective on life and how I do things. I also felt that I was able to love Hope in a deeper way after being exposed to the love that giving birth brought to me. I loved her with all of my heart already; Jayden's birth just gave me a rekindled love and appreciation for my darling daughter.

I was absolutely thrilled with my labor and delivery experience. I never pass up an opportunity to share it with someone to encourage them or just to reminisce. I felt like I progressed quickly for my first birth and that every aspect of pain that I had was manageable. I pride myself in gloating that I didn't scream once. It was my hidden fear that I would be a maniac as I tried to deal with my labor. I was most ecstatic that my epidural "kicked in," giving me a pain-free delivery.

God blessed me tremendously as He answered my father-in-law's prayer for me to have a quick, safe and painless delivery. I felt extremely blessed by the fact that Jayden was perfect and healthy despite all of the complications that arose during my pregnancy and labor. God has been so incredible. I am overwhelmed by His love for me and my family. God certainly was not obligated to answer our prayers, but He did. I have felt so unworthy of the love and compassion God has shown me.

We took our angel baby home on May 12, 2001 and celebrated my first official Mother's Day the next morning. We encountered a few bumps in the road, which did not surprise us. I developed a fever shortly after being home. I was treated with antibiotics just to be safe. Also, it seemed I had sustained a broken tailbone during delivery that still gives me pain. Otherwise, my recovery went very well.

On July 6, 2001, Hope's second adoption anniversary, we dedicated Jayden to the Lord. It was a very reverent service as we celebrated the miracle God so graciously bestowed upon us. Jody's father and my father spoke at the service, proclaiming God's goodness and faithfulness by giving us our special gift. Afterward, we pledged vows stating we would raise Jayden for the Lord and by His word.

We watched a presentation that Jody's parents put together from pictures and video segments that we had already collected of our newborn. They set it to music that was profoundly appropriate. As pictures of my pregnancy and labor lit up the screen, a song explained them with its lyrics, "Waiting on you, I'm patiently waiting on you." When pictures of Jayden's birth appeared, the Hallelujah chorus rang out. Another song proclaimed that "Nothing at all is impossible for God" while clips of our miracle baby danced on the screen before us. It was a fabulous presentation capturing our forever memories. Jody also sang the song I wrote for Jayden several years ago while waiting for him:

"Angel Baby"

Verse 1—As a man and a woman, we had a great desire. So we withstood the tests and impossibilities, but grew troubled and very tired. You see, we were told we'd live a solitary life. It would be a home without a child, just a husband and a wife. So we prayed...

Chorus—From our lips to heaven's ears, we called you from afar. God heard, then gently spoke the word. Now here you are! From our lips to heaven's ears. Our desire He has filled. You're the miracle of miracles! God placed you in our arms.

Verse 2—Oh, the angels up in heaven must have shed a tear that day. When God announced their treasure soon would go away. You

132

would leave heaven's glory to longing hearts below. Just to prove His faithfulness and the love He shows. Because we prayed... (Repeat chorus)

I felt so humbled that I was given a marvelous gift like Jayden and so indebted to God for His kind favor upon me. We continued to give thanks to God and celebrated the most remarkable event of my life.

Everyday with Jayden has been like our first day together. There is always something new to experience and something new to discover about him. Sometimes the simplest thing he does brings such astonishment to us. I have found motherhood to cause such an awakening in me. It is the most awesome and wonderful thing I could ever imagine. I soak up every little accomplishment Jayden makes as if he just performed an unbelievable feat. I can't imagine life without him now, and even more, I can't imagine someone going through life not being able to have this for themselves. That thought absolutely crushes me. Jayden is the most gentle, pleasant and angelic baby I have ever met. I have no doubt that his precious life has a special purpose. I can already sense it as I gaze into those deep, thoughtful eyes. At times he gives me the feeling that he knows more about his presence than I do while he stares intently into my eyes.

I still wear a jagged scar over my heart that resulted from the ugly wound infertility created within. The pain from my trauma is lessened, but that area of my heart remains "sore." Each time I revisit the darker moments of my life and the trials of my faith, the pain wells up within me and I often weep. I become broken, realizing how God reached down and pulled me out of my calamity to answer my prayer, giving me my miracle. In all of His infinite power and glory, He simply reached out His hand of mercy and gave me my baby—my miracle.

When I meet or talk with someone who is struggling with infertility it brushes against that tender scar, sending twinges of pain through my heart for her. I become emotional remembering the desolation I felt, the helplessness, and the indescribable pain that was my unwelcome companion during that time in my life. That pain has been replaced by a burden in my heart for those who have not been privileged to conceive. I do my best to encourage them, share my testimony, and seek God with fasting and prayer in their behalf as I relate to their struggle and very real pain that they are trying to cope with.

Jayden's life has already been a testimony to those couples and others around us. I make it a point to tell everyone we meet that he is our miracle from God. I go on to say that it took many prayers to get him here. I like to attest to the fact that God still performs miracles and does answer prayers. After all, He answered mine!

As memories fade and my story becomes old, the legacy of the miracle God gave me will carry on. Because every time someone calls Jayden's name, it gives glory to God for answering our prayers as the meaning of his name testifies and confirms: "Jehovah has heard."